Virtual Clinical Excursions—

for

Fortinash and Holoday Worret: Psychiatric Mental Health Nursing, 4th Edition

prepared by

Susan Fertig McDonald, MSN, RN, CS, DNP(c)
Clinical Nurse Specialist—Psychiatry
VA San Diego Healthcare System
San Diego, California

software developed by

Wolfsong Informatics, LLC
Tucson, Arizona

MOSBY
ELSEVIER

MOSBY
ELSEVIER

11830 Westline Industrial Dr.
St. Louis, Missouri 63146

VIRTUAL CLINICAL EXCURSIONS—PSYCHIATRIC FOR
FORTINASH AND HOLODAY WORRET:
PSYCHIATRIC MENTAL HEALTH NURSING
FOURTH EDITION

ISBN: 978-0-323-05012-8

Notice

Knowledge and best practice in this field are constantly changing. As new research and experience broaden our knowledge, changes in practice, treatment and drug therapy may become necessary or appropriate. Readers are advised to check the most current information provided (i) on procedures featured or (ii) by the manufacturer of each product to be administered, to verify the recommended dose or formula, the method and duration of administration, and contraindications. It is the responsibility of the practitioner, relying on their own experience and knowledge of the patient, to make diagnoses, to determine dosages and the best treatment for each individual patient, and to take all appropriate safety precautions. To the fullest extent of the law, neither the Publisher nor the Authors assumes any liability for any injury and/or damage to persons or property arising out or related to any use of the material contained in this book.

ISBN: 978-0-323-05012-8

Executive Publisher, Nursing: *Tom Wilhelm*
Managing Editor: *Jeff Downing*
Associate Developmental Editor: *Tiffany Trautwein*
Book Production Manager: *Gayle May*
Project Manager: *Tracey Schriefer*

Printed in the United States of America

Last digit is the print number: 9 8 7 6 5 4

Workbook
prepared by

Susan Fertig McDonald, MSN, RN, CS, DNP(c)
Clinical Nurse Specialist—Psychiatry
VA San Diego Healthcare System
San Diego, California

Textbook

Katherine M. Fortinash, MSN, APRN, BC
Certified Clinical Specialist
Adult Psychiatric-Mental Health Nursing;
Associate Faculty
Mt. San Jacinto College
Menifee, California;
Clinical Nurse Specialist and Educator
Sharp Healthcare, Mesa Vista Hospital
San Diego, California;

Patricia A. Holoday Worret, MSN, APRN, BC
Certified Clinical Specialist
Adult Psychiatric Mental Health Nursing;
Professor, Psychiatric Mental Health Nursing
Palomar College
San Marcos, California;
Consultant
San Diego, California

Reviewer

Carissa Enright, MSN, RN
Clinical Assistant Professor
Nursing Faculty, College of Nursing
Texas Woman's University
Dallas, Texas

Contents

Getting Started

Lessons

Table of Contents
Fortinash and Holoday Worret:
Psychiatric Mental Health Nursing, 4th Edition

Getting Started

GETTING SET UP

MINIMUM SYSTEM REQUIREMENTS

Windows®

Windows Vista™, XP, 2000 (Recommend Windows XP/2000)
Pentium® III processor (or equivalent) @ 600 MHz (Recommend 800 MHz or better)
256 MB of RAM (Recommend 1 GB or more for Windows Vista)
800 x 600 screen size (Recommend 1024 x 768)
Thousands of colors
12x CD-ROM drive
Soundblaster 16 soundcard compatibility
Stereo speakers or headphones

Note: Windows Vista and XP require administrator privileges for installation.

Macintosh®

MAC OS X (10.2 or higher)
Apple Power PC G3 @ 500 MHz or better
128 MB of RAM (Recommend 256 MB or more)
800 x 600 screen size (Recommend 1024 x 768)
Thousands of colors
12x CD-ROM drive
Stereo speakers or headphones

■ INSTALLATION INSTRUCTIONS

WINDOWS

1. Insert the *Virtual Clinical Excursions—Psychiatric* CD-ROM.
2. The setup screen should appear automatically if the current product is not already installed. Windows Vista users may be asked to authorize additional security prompts.
3. Follow the onscreen instructions during the setup process.

If the setup screen does *not* appear automatically (and *Virtual Clinical Excursions—Psychiatric* has not been installed already):

a. Click the **My Computer** icon on your desktop or on your Start menu.
b. Double-click on your CD-ROM drive.
c. If installation does not start at this point:
   (1) Click the **Start** icon on the taskbar and select the **Run** option.
   (2) Type d:\setup.exe (where "d:\" is your CD-ROM drive) and press **OK**.
   (3) Follow the onscreen instructions for installation.

MACINTOSH

1. Insert the *Virtual Clinical Excursions—Psychiatric* CD in the CD-ROM drive. The disk icon will appear on your desktop.
2. Double-click on the disk icon.
3. Double-click on the PSYCHIATRIC_MAC run file.

Note: Virtual Clinical Excursions—Psychiatric for Macintosh does not have an installation setup and can only be run directly from the CD.

■ HOW TO USE VIRTUAL CLINICAL EXCURSIONS—PSYCHIATRIC

WINDOWS

1. Double-click on the *Virtual Clinical Excursions—Psychiatric* icon located on your desktop.
2. Or navigate to the program via the Windows Start menu.

Note: If your computer uses Windows Vista, right-click on the desktop shortcut and choose **Properties**. In the Compatability Mode, check the box for "Run as Administrator." Below is a screen capture to show what this looks like.

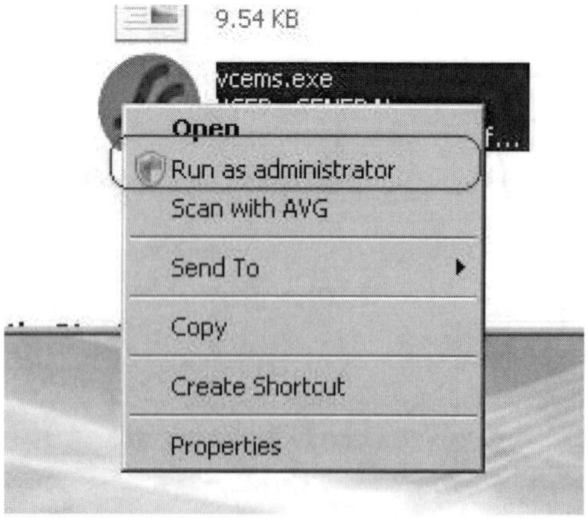

MACINTOSH

1. Insert the *Virtual Clinical Excursions—Psychiatric* CD in the CD-ROM drive. The disk icon will appear on your desktop.
2. Double-click on the disk icon.
3. Double-click on the PSYCHIATRIC_MAC run file.

SCREEN SETTINGS

For best results, your computer monitor resolution should be set at a minimum of 800 x 600. The number of colors displayed should be set to "thousands or higher" (High Color or 16 bit) or "millions of colors" (True Color or 24 bit).

Windows

1. From the **Start** menu, select **Control Panel** (on some systems, you will first go to **Settings**, then to **Control Panel**).
2. Double-click on the **Display** icon.
3. Click on the **Settings** tab.
4. Under **Screen resolution** use the slider bar to select **800 by 600 pixels**.
5. Access the **Colors** drop-down menu by clicking on the down arrow.
6. Select **High Color (16 bit)** or **True Color (24 bit)**.
7. Click on **OK**.
8. You may be asked to verify the setting changes. Click **Yes**.
9. You may be asked to restart your computer to accept the changes. Click **Yes**.

Macintosh

1. Select the **Monitors** control panel.
2. Select **800 x 600** (or similar) from the **Resolution** area.
3. Select **Thousands** or **Millions** from the **Color Depth** area.

WEB BROWSERS

Supported web browsers include Microsoft Internet Explorer (IE) version 6.0 or higher and Mozilla Firefox version 2.0 or higher. The supported browser for Macs running OS X is Mozilla Firefox.

If you use America Online® (AOL) for web access, you will need AOL version 4.0 or higher and one of the browsers listed above. Do not use earlier versions of AOL with earlier versions of IE, because you will have difficulty accessing many features.

For best results with AOL:

- Connect to the Internet using AOL version 4.0 or higher.
- Open a private chat within AOL (this allows the AOL client to remain open, without asking whether you wish to disconnect while minimized).
- Minimize AOL.
- Launch a recommended browser.

TECHNICAL SUPPORT

Technical support for this product is available between 7:30 a.m. and 7 p.m. (CST), Monday through Friday. Before calling, be sure that your computer meets the minimum system requirements to run this software. Inside the United States and Canada, call 1-800-692-9010. Outside North America, call 314-872-8370. You may also fax your questions to 314-523-4932 or contact Technical Support through e-mail: technical.support@elsevier.com.

Trademarks: Windows, Macintosh, Pentium, and America Online are registered trademarks.

ACCESSING *Virtual Clinical Excursions—Psychiatric* FROM EVOLVE

The product you have purchased is part of the Evolve family of online courses and learning resources. Please read the following information thoroughly to get started.

To access your instructor's course on Evolve:

Your instructor will provide you with the username and password needed to access this specific course on the Evolve Learning System. Once you have received this information, please follow these instructions:

1. Go to the Evolve student page (http://evolve.elsevier.com/student).
2. Enter your username and password in the **Login to My Evolve** area and click the **Login** button.
3. You will be taken to your personalized **My Evolve** page, where the course will be listed in the **My Courses** module.

TECHNICAL REQUIREMENTS

To use an Evolve course, you will need access to a computer that is connected to the Internet and equipped with web browser software that supports frames. For optimal performance, it is recommended that you have speakers and use a high-speed Internet connection. However, slower dial-up modems (56 K minimum) are acceptable.

Whichever browser you use, the browser preferences must be set to enable cookies and JavaScript and the cache must be set to reload every time.

Enable Cookies

Browser	Steps
Internet Explorer (IE) 6.0 or higher	**1.** Select **Tools → Internet Options**. **2.** Select **Privacy** tab. **3.** Use the slider (slide down) to **Accept All Cookies**. **4.** Click **OK**. **-OR-** **3.** Click the **Advanced** button. **4.** Click the check box next to **Override Automatic Cookie Handling**. **5.** Click the **Accept** radio buttons under **First-party Cookies** and **Third-party Cookies**. **6.** Click **OK**.
Mozilla Firefox 2.0 or higher	**1.** Select **Tools → Options**. **2.** Select the **Privacy** icon. **3.** Click to expand Cookies. **4.** Select **Allow sites to set cookies**. **5.** Click **OK**.

Set Cache to Always Reload a Page

Browser	Steps
Internet Explorer (IE) 6.0 or higher	**1.** Select **Tools → Internet Options**. **2.** Select **General** tab. **3.** Go to the **Temporary Internet Files** and click the **Settings** button. **4.** Select the radio button for **Every visit to the page** and click **OK** when complete.
Mozilla Firefox 2.0 or higher	**1.** Select **Tools → Options**. **2.** Select the **Privacy** icon. **3.** Click to expand Cache. **4.** Set the value to "**0**" in the **Use up to: __ MB of disk space for the cache** field. **5.** Click **OK**.

Plug-Ins

Adobe Acrobat Reader—With the free Acrobat Reader software, you can view and print Adobe PDF files. Many Evolve products offer student and instructor manuals, checklists, and more in this format!

Download at: http://www.adobe.com

Apple QuickTime—Install this to hear word pronunciations, heart and lung sounds, and many other helpful audio clips within Evolve Online Courses!

Download at: http://www.apple.com

Adobe Flash Player—This player will enhance your viewing of many Evolve web pages, as well as educational short-form to long-form animation within the Evolve Learning System!

Download at: http://www.adobe.com

Adobe Shockwave Player—Shockwave is best for viewing the many interactive learning activities within Evolve Online Courses!

Download at: http://www.adobe.com

Microsoft Word Viewer—With this viewer, Microsoft Word users can share documents with those who don't have Word, and users without Word can open and view Word documents. Many Evolve products have testbank, student and instructor manuals, and other documents available for downloading and viewing on your own computer!

Download at: http://www.microsoft.com

Microsoft PowerPoint Viewer—With this viewer, you can access PowerPoint 97, 2000, and 2002 presentations even if you don't have PowerPoint. Many Evolve products have slides available for downloading and viewing on your own computer!

Download at: http://www.microsoft.com

SUPPORT INFORMATION

Live phone support is available to customers in the United States and Canada at **800-401-9962** from 7:30 a.m. to 7 p.m. (CST), Monday through Friday. Support is also available through email at evolve-support@elsevier.com.

Online 24/7 support can be accessed on the Evolve website (http://evolve.elsevier.com). Resources include:

- Guided tours
- Tutorials
- Frequently asked questions (FAQs)
- Online copies of course user guides
- And much more!

A QUICK TOUR

Welcome to *Virtual Clinical Excursions—Psychiatric*, a virtual hospital setting in which you can work with multiple complex patient simulations and also learn to access and evaluate the information resources that are essential for high-quality patient care. The virtual hospital, Pacific View Regional Hospital, has realistic architecture and access to patient rooms, a Nurses' Station, and a Medication Room.

BEFORE YOU START

Make sure you have your textbook nearby when you use the *Virtual Clinical Excursions—Psychiatric* CD. You will want to consult topic areas in your textbook frequently while working with the CD and using this workbook.

HOW TO SIGN IN

- Enter your name on the Student Nurse identification badge.
- Next, click the down arrow next to **Select Floor**. This drop-down menu lists only the floors on which there are currently patients with psychiatric nursing needs: Medical-Surgical, Obstetrics, Pediatrics, and Skilled Nursing. (For this quick tour, choose **Obstetrics**.)
- Now choose one of the four periods of care in which to work. In Periods of Care 1 through 3, you can actively engage in patient assessment, entry of data in the electronic patient record (EPR), and medication administration. Period of Care 4 presents the day in review. Highlight and click the appropriate period of care. (For this quick tour, choose **Period of Care 1**.)
- Click **Go**. This takes you to the Patient List screen (see example on page 11). Note that the virtual time is provided in the box at the lower left corner of the screen (0730, since we chose Period of Care 1).

Note: If you choose to work during Period of Care 4: 1900-2000, the Patient List screen is skipped since you are not able to visit patients or administer medications during the shift. Instead, you are taken directly to the Nurses' Station, where the records of all the patients on the floor are available for your review.

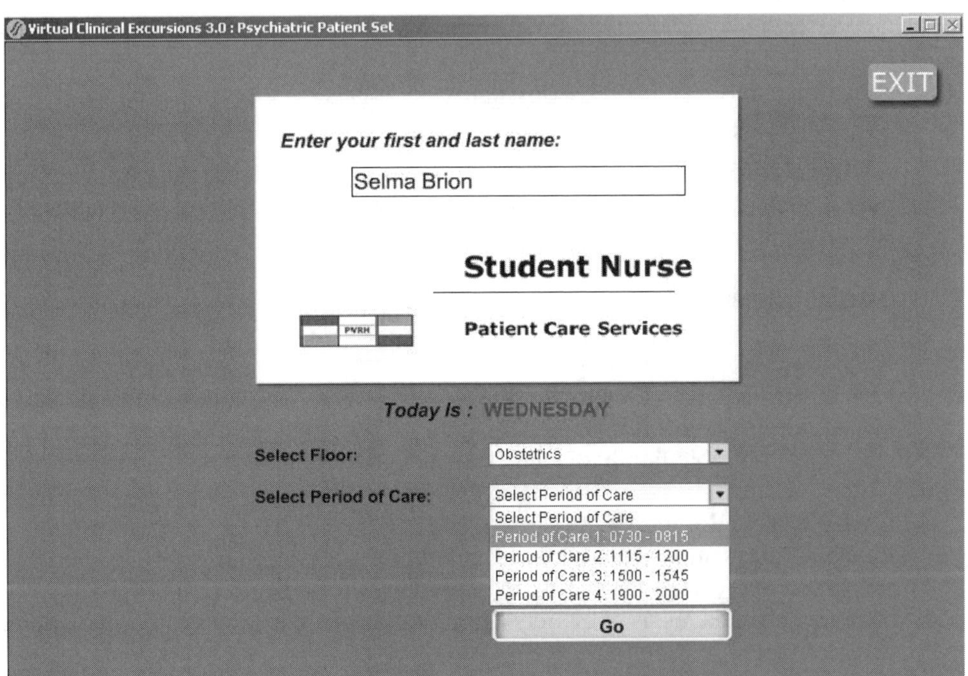

PATIENT LIST

OBSTETRICS UNIT

Dorothy Grant (Room 201)
30-week intrauterine pregnancy—A 25-year-old Caucasian multipara admitted with abdominal trauma following a domestic violence incident. Her complications include preterm labor and extensive social issues such as acquiring safe housing for her family upon discharge.

Kelly Brady (Room 203)
26-week intrauterine pregnancy—A 35-year-old Caucasian primigravida urgently admitted for progressive symptoms of preeclampsia. A history of inadequate coping with major life stressors leave her at risk for a recurrence of depression as she faces a diagnosis of HELLP syndrome and the delivery of a severely premature infant.

Laura Wilson (Room 206)
37-week intrauterine pregnancy—An 18-year-old Caucasian primigravida urgently admitted after being found unconscious. Her complications include HIV-positive status and chronic polysubstance abuse. Unrealistic expectations of parenthood and living with a chronic illness, combined with strained family relations, prompt comprehensive social and psychiatric evaluations initiated on the day of simulation.

PEDIATRIC UNIT

Tiffany Sheldon (Room 305)
Anorexia nervosa—A 14-year-old Caucasian female admitted for dehydration, electrolyte imbalance, and malnutrition following a syncope episode at home. This patient has a history of eating disorders that have required multiple hospital admissions and have strained family dynamics between mother and daughter.

MEDICAL-SURGICAL UNIT

Harry George (Room 401)
Osteomyelitis—A 54-year-old Caucasian male admitted from a homeless shelter with an infected leg. He has complications of type 2 diabetes mellitus, alcohol abuse, nicotine addiction, poor pain control, and complex psychosocial issues.

Jacquline Catanazaro (Room 402)
Asthma—A 45-year-old Caucasian female admitted with an acute asthma exacerbation and suspected pneumonia. She has complications of chronic schizophrenia, noncompliance with medication therapy, obesity, and herniated disk.

SKILLED NURSING UNIT

Kathryn Doyle (Room 503)
Rehabilitation post left hip replacement—A 79-year-old Caucasian female admitted following a complicated recovery from an ORIF. She is experiencing symptoms of malnutrition and depression due to unstable family dynamics, placing her at risk for elder abuse.

Carlos Reyes (Room 504)
Rehabilitation status post myocardial infarction—An 81-year-old Hispanic male admitted for evaluation of the need for long-term care following an acute care hospital stay. Recent cognitive changes and a diagnosis of anxiety disorder contribute to stressful family dynamics and caregiver strain.

HOW TO SELECT A PATIENT

- You can choose one or more patients to work with from the Patient List by checking the box to the left of the patient name(s). For this quick tour, select Dorothy Grant. (In order to receive a scorecard for a patient, the patient must be selected before proceeding to the Nurses' Station.)
- Click on **Get Report** to the right of the medical records number (MRN) to view a summary of the patient's care during the 12-hour period before your arrival on the unit.
- After reviewing the report, click on **Go to Nurses' Station** in the right lower corner to begin your care. (*Note:* If you have been assigned to care for multiple patients, you can click on **Return to Patient List** to select and review the report for each additional patient before going to the Nurses' Station.)

Note: Even though the Patient List is initially skipped when you sign in to work for Period of Care 4, you can still access this screen if you wish to review the shift report for any of the patients. To do so, simply click on **Patient List** near the top left corner of the Nurses' Station (or click on the clipboard to the left of the Kardex). Then click on **Get Report** for the patient(s) whose care you are reviewing. This may be done during any period of care.

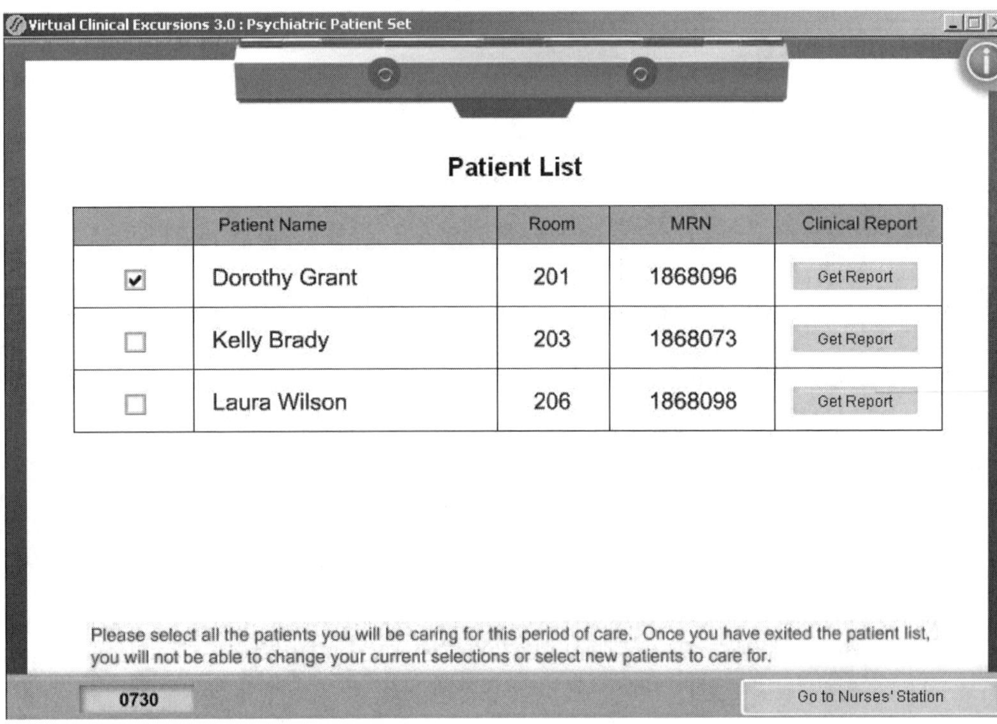

HOW TO FIND A PATIENT'S RECORDS

NURSES' STATION

Within the Nurses' Station, you will see:

1. A clipboard that contains the patient list for that floor.
2. A chart rack with patient charts labeled by room number, a notebook labeled Kardex, and a notebook labeled MAR (Medication Administration Record).
3. A desktop computer with access to the Electronic Patient Record (EPR).
4. A tool bar across the top of the screen that can also be used to access the Patient List, EPR, Chart, MAR, and Kardex. This tool bar is also accessible from each patient's room.
5. A Drug Guide containing information about the medications you are able to administer to your patients.
6. A tool bar across the bottom of the screen that can be used to access the Floor Map, patient rooms, Medication Room, and Drug Guide.

As you run your cursor over an item, it will be highlighted. To select, simply double-click on the item. As you use these resources, you will always be able to return to the Nurses' Station by clicking on the **Return to Nurses' Station** bar located in the right lower corner of your screen.

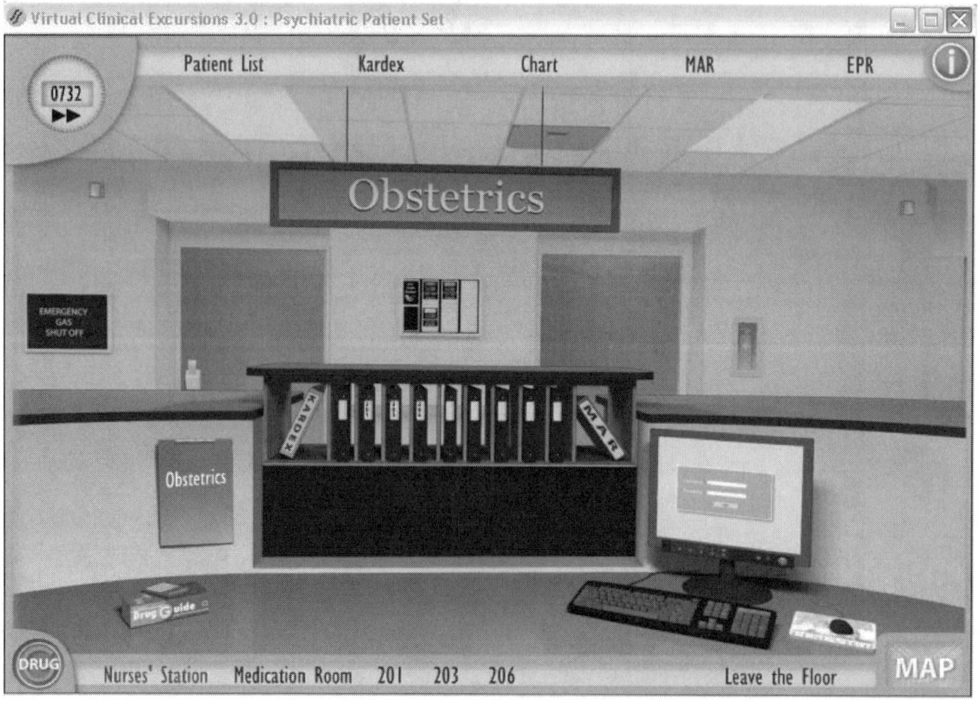

MEDICATION ADMINISTRATION RECORD (MAR)

The MAR icon located on the tool bar at the top of your screen accesses current 24-hour medications for each patient. Click on the icon and the MAR will open. (*Note:* You can also access the MAR by clicking on the MAR notebook on the far right side of the book rack in the center of the screen.) Within the MAR, tabs on the right side of the screen allow you to select patients by room number. Be careful to make sure you select the correct tab number for *your* patient rather than simply reading the first record that appears after the MAR opens. Each MAR sheet lists the following:

- Medications
- Route and dosage of each medication
- Times of administration of each medication

Note: The MAR changes each day. Expired MARs are stored in the patients' charts.

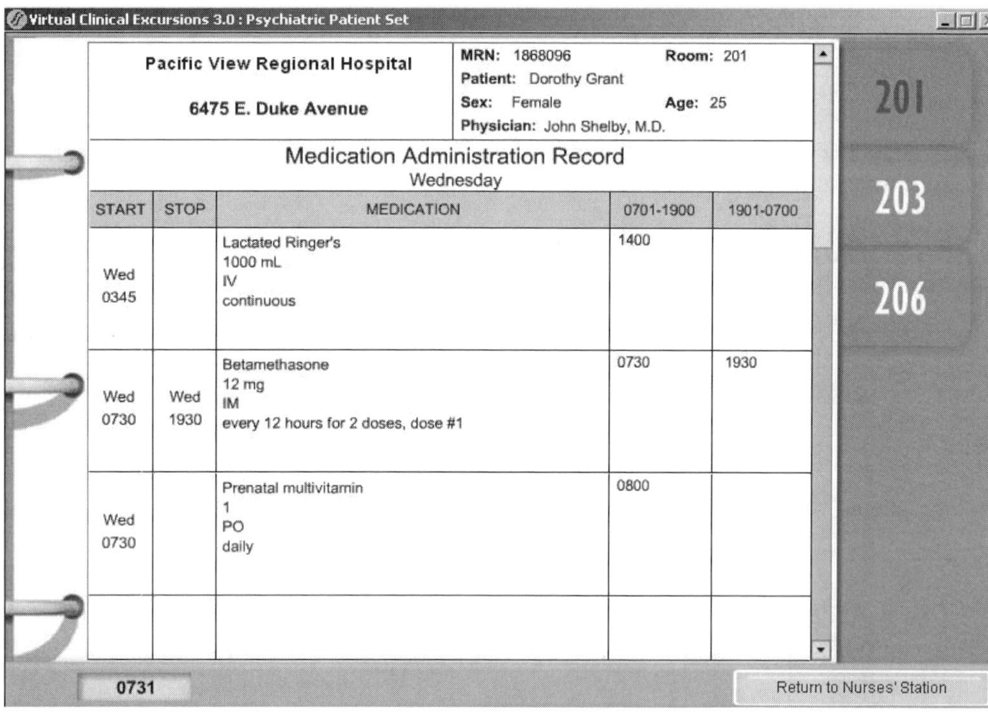

CHARTS

To access patient charts, either click on the **Chart** icon at the top of your screen or anywhere within the chart rack in the center of the Nurses' Station screen. When the close-up view appears, the individual charts are labeled by room number. To open a chart, click on the room number of the patient whose chart you wish to review. The patient's name and allergies will appear on the left side of the screen, along with a list of tabs on the right side of the screen, allowing you to view the following data:

- Allergies
- Physician's Orders
- Physician's Notes
- Nurse's Notes
- Laboratory Reports
- Diagnostic Reports
- Surgical Reports
- Consultations
- Patient Education
- History and Physical
- Nursing Admission
- Expired MARs
- Consents
- Mental Health
- Admissions
- Emergency Department

Information appears in real time. The entries are in reverse chronologic order, so use the down arrow at the right side of each chart page to scroll down to view previous entries. Flip from tab to tab to view multiple data fields or click on **Return to Nurses' Station** in the lower right corner of the screen to exit the chart.

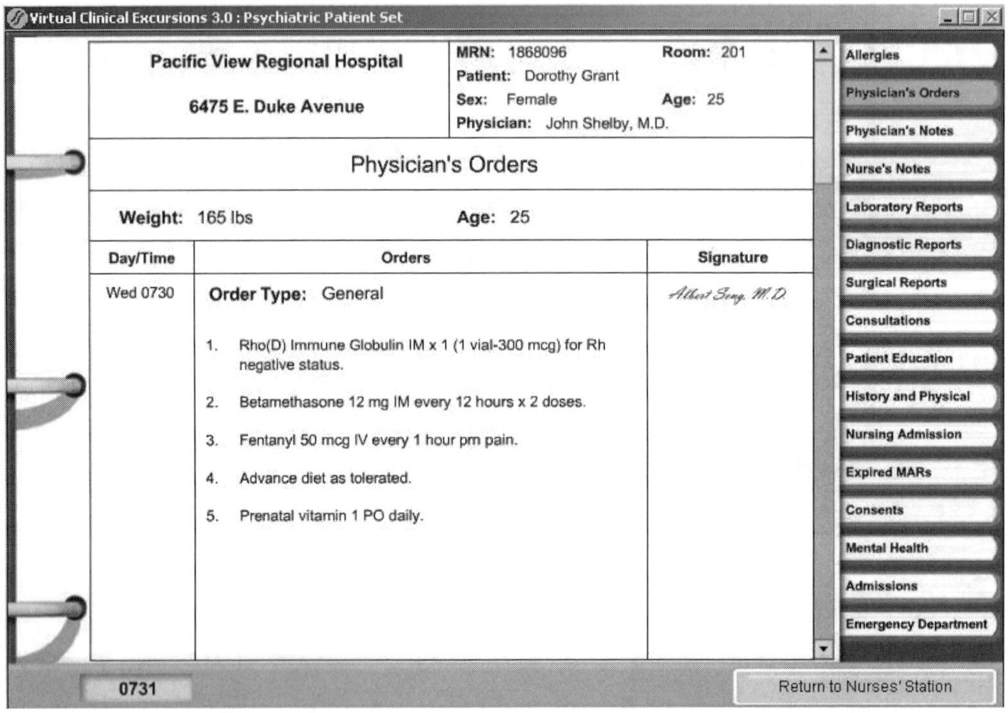

Electronic Patient Record (EPR)

The EPR can be accessed from the computer in the Nurses' Station or from the EPR icon located in the tool bar at the top of your screen. To access a patient's EPR:

- Click on either the computer screen or the **EPR** icon.
- Your username and password are automatically filled in.
- Click on **Login** to enter the EPR.
- *Note:* Like the MAR, the EPR is arranged numerically. Thus when you enter, you are initially shown the records of the patient in the lowest room number on the floor. To view the correct data for *your* patient, remember to select the correct room number, using the drop-down menu for the Patient field at the top left corner of the screen.

The EPR used in Pacific View Regional Hospital represents a composite of commercial versions being used in hospitals. You can access the EPR:

- to review existing data for a patient (by room number).
- to enter data you collect while working with a patient.

The EPR is updated daily, so no matter what day or part of a shift you are working, there will be a current EPR with the patient's data from the past days of the current hospital stay. This type of simulated EPR allows you to examine how data for different attributes have changed over time, as well as to examine data for all of a patient's attributes at a particular time. The EPR is fully functional (as it is in a real-life hospital). You can enter such data as blood pressure, breath sounds, and certain treatments. The EPR will not, however, allow you to enter data for a previous time period. Use the arrows at the bottom of the screen to move forward and backward in time.

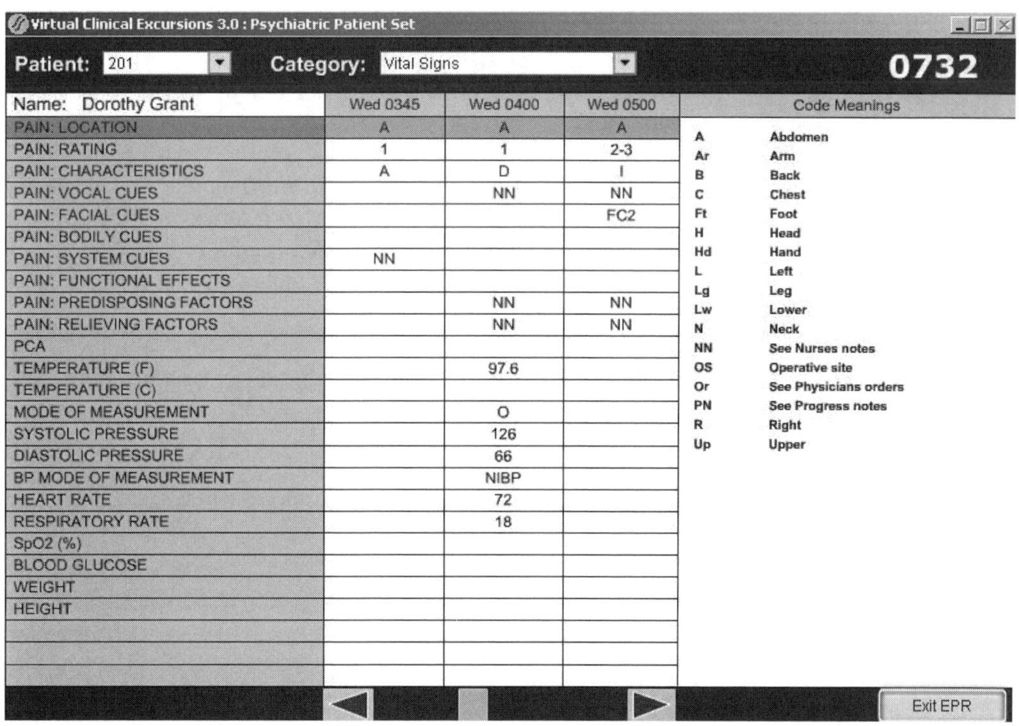

Virtual Clinical Excursions 3.0 : Psychiatric Patient Set

Patient: 201 Category: Vital Signs 0732

Name: Dorothy Grant	Wed 0345	Wed 0400	Wed 0500
PAIN: LOCATION	A	A	A
PAIN: RATING	1	1	2-3
PAIN: CHARACTERISTICS	A	D	I
PAIN: VOCAL CUES		NN	NN
PAIN: FACIAL CUES			FC2
PAIN: BODILY CUES			
PAIN: SYSTEM CUES	NN		
PAIN: FUNCTIONAL EFFECTS			
PAIN: PREDISPOSING FACTORS		NN	NN
PAIN: RELIEVING FACTORS		NN	NN
PCA			
TEMPERATURE (F)		97.6	
TEMPERATURE (C)			
MODE OF MEASUREMENT		O	
SYSTOLIC PRESSURE		126	
DIASTOLIC PRESSURE		66	
BP MODE OF MEASUREMENT		NIBP	
HEART RATE		72	
RESPIRATORY RATE		18	
SpO2 (%)			
BLOOD GLUCOSE			
WEIGHT			
HEIGHT			

Code Meanings	
A	Abdomen
Ar	Arm
B	Back
C	Chest
Ft	Foot
H	Head
Hd	Hand
L	Left
Lg	Leg
Lw	Lower
N	Neck
NN	See Nurses notes
OS	Operative site
Or	See Physicians orders
PN	See Progress notes
R	Right
Up	Upper

Exit EPR

At the top of the EPR screen, you can choose patients by their room numbers. In addition, you have access to 17 different categories of patient data. To change patients or data categories, click the down arrow to the right of the room number or category.

The categories of patient data in the EPR as as follows:

- Vital Signs
- Respiratory
- Cardiovascular
- Neurologic
- Gastrointestinal
- Excretory
- Musculoskeletal
- Integumentary
- Reproductive
- Psychosocial
- Wounds and Drains
- Activity
- Hygiene and Comfort
- Safety
- Nutrition
- IV
- Intake and Output

Remember, each hospital selects its own codes. The codes used in the EPR at Pacific View Regional Hospital may be different from ones you have seen in your clinical rotations. Take some time to acquaint yourself with the codes. Within the Vital Signs category, click on any item in the left column (e.g., Pain: Characteristics). In the far-right column, you will see a list of code meanings for the possible findings and/or descriptors for that assessment area.

You will use the codes to record the data you collect as you work with patients. Click on the box in the last time column to the right of any item and wait for the code meanings applicable to that entry to appear. Select the appropriate code to describe your assessment findings and type it in the box. (*Note:* If no cursor appears within the box, click on the box again until the blue shading disappears and the blinking cursor appears.) Once the data are typed in this box, they are entered into the patient's record for this period of care only.

To leave the EPR, click on **Exit EPR** in the bottom right corner of the screen.

VISITING A PATIENT

From the Nurses' Station, click on the room number of the patient you wish to visit (in the tool bar at the bottom of your screen). Once you are inside the room, you will see a still photo of your patient in the top left corner. To verify that this is the correct patient, click on the **Check Armband** icon to the right of the photo. The patient's identification data will appear. If you click on **Check Allergies** (the next icon to the right), a list of the patient's allergies (if any) will replace the photo.

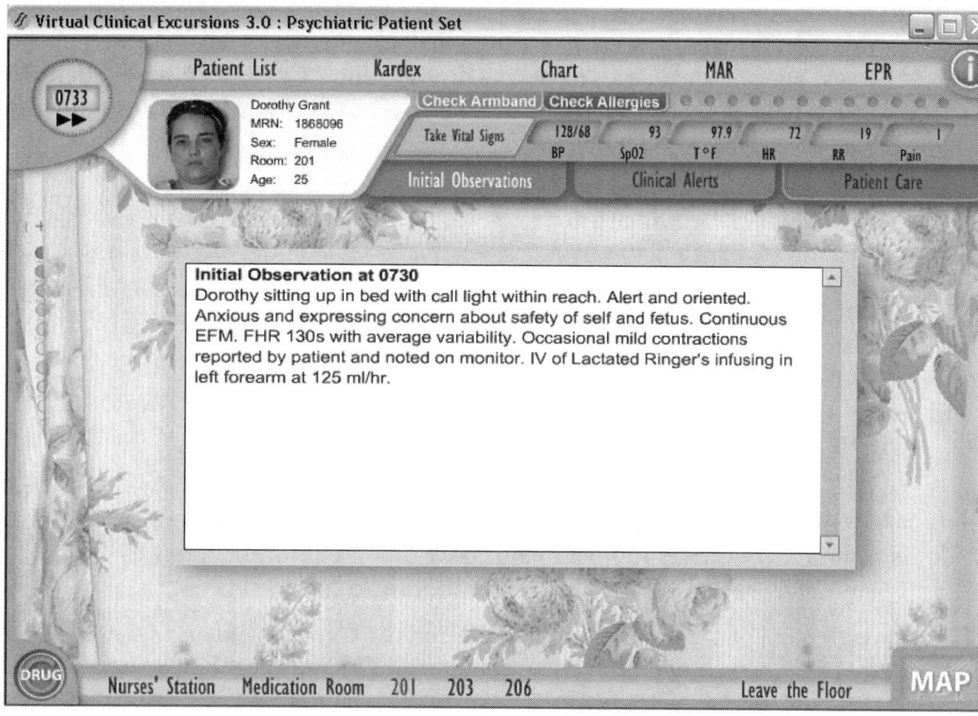

Also located in the patient's room are multiple icons you can use to assess the patient or the patient's medications. A virtual clock is provided in the upper left corner of the room to monitor your progress in real time. (*Note:* The fast-forward icon within the virtual clock will advance the time by 2-minute intervals when clicked.)

- The tool bar across the top of the screen allows you to check the **Patient List**, access the **EPR** to check or enter data, and view the patient's **Chart**, **MAR**, or **Kardex**.
- The **Take Vital Signs** icon allows you to measure the patient's up-to-the-minute blood pressure, oxygen saturation, temperature, heart rate, respiratory rate, and pain level.
- Each time you enter a patient's room, you are given an Initial Observation report to review (in the text box under the patient's photo). These notes are provided to give you a "look" at the patient as if you had just stepped into the room. You can also click on the **Initial Observations** icon to return to this box from other views within the patient's room. To the right of this icon is **Clinical Alerts**, a resource that allows you to make decisions about priority medication interventions based on emerging data collected in real time. Check this screen throughout your period of care to avoid missing critical information related to recently ordered or STAT medications.
- Clicking on **Patient Care** opens up three specific learning environments within the patient room: **Physical Assessment**, **Nurse-Client Interactions**, and **Medication Administration**.
- To perform a **Physical Assessment**, choose a body area (such as **Head & Neck**) from the column of yellow buttons. This activates a list of system subcategories for that body area (e.g., see **Sensory**, **Neurologic**, etc. in the green boxes). After you select the system you

wish to evaluate, a brief description of the assessment findings will appear in a box to the right. A still photo provides a "snapshot" of how an assessment of this area might be done or what the finding might look like. For every body area, you can also click on **Equipment** on the right side of the screen.

- To the right of the Physical Assessment icon is **Nurse-Client Interactions**. Clicking on this icon will reveal the times and titles of any videos available for viewing. (*Note:* If the video you wish to see is not listed, this means you have not yet reached the correct virtual time to view that video. Check the virtual clock; you may return to access the video once its designated time has occurred—as long as you do so within the same period of care. Or you can click on the fast-forward icon within the virtual clock to advance the time by 2-minute intervals. You will then need to click again on **Patient Care** and **Nurse-Client Interactions** to refresh the screen.) To view a listed video, click on the white arrow to the right of the video title. Use the control buttons below the video to start, stop, pause, rewind, or fast-forward the action or to mute the sound.
- **Medication Administration** is the pathway that allows you to review and administer medications to a patient after you have prepared them in the Medication Room. This process is addressed further in the *How to Prepare Medications* section (pages 19-20) and in *Medications* (pages 26-30). For additional hands-on practice, see *Reducing Medication Errors* (pages 37-41).

HOW TO QUIT, CHANGE PATIENTS, CHANGE FLOORS, OR CHANGE PERIODS OF CARE

How to Quit: From most screens, you may click the **Leave the Floor** icon on the bottom tool bar to the right of the patient room numbers. (*Note:* From some screens, you will first need to click an **Exit** button or **Return to Nurses' Station** before clicking **Leave the Floor**.) When the Floor Menu appears, click **Exit** to leave the program.

How to Change Patients, Floors, or Periods of Care: To change patients, simply click on the new patient's room number. (You cannot receive a scorecard for a new patient, however, unless you have already selected that patient on the Patient List screen.) To change to a new period of care, to change floors, or to restart the virtual clock, click on **Leave the Floor** and then on **Restart the Program**.

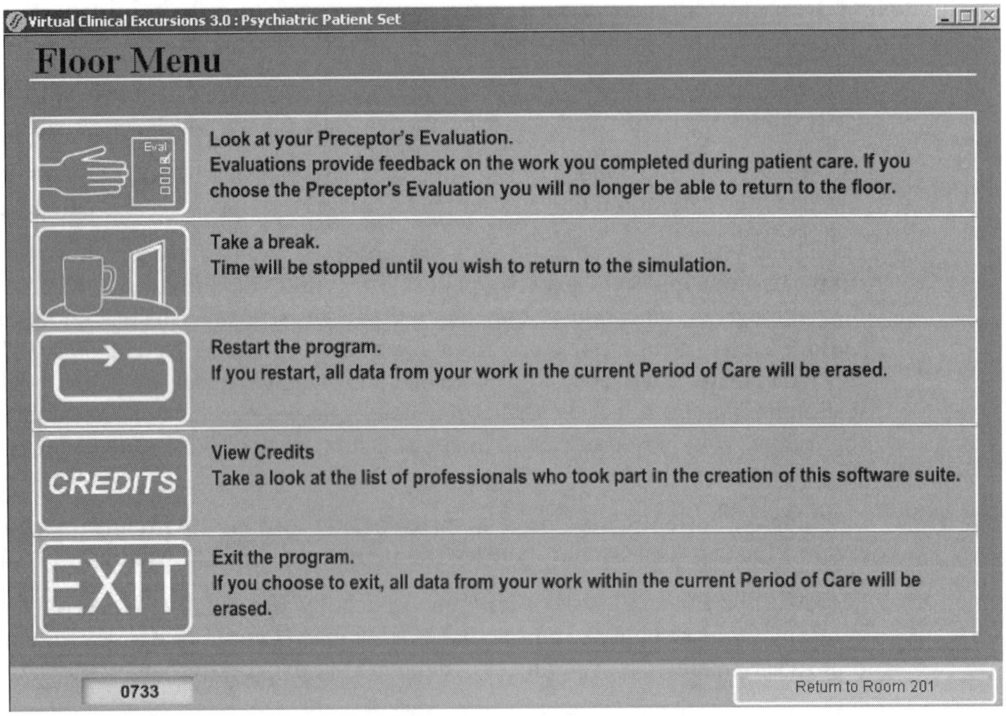

HOW TO PREPARE MEDICATIONS

From the Nurses' Station or the patient's room, you can access the Medication Room by clicking on the icon in the tool bar at the bottom of your screen to the left of the patient room numbers.

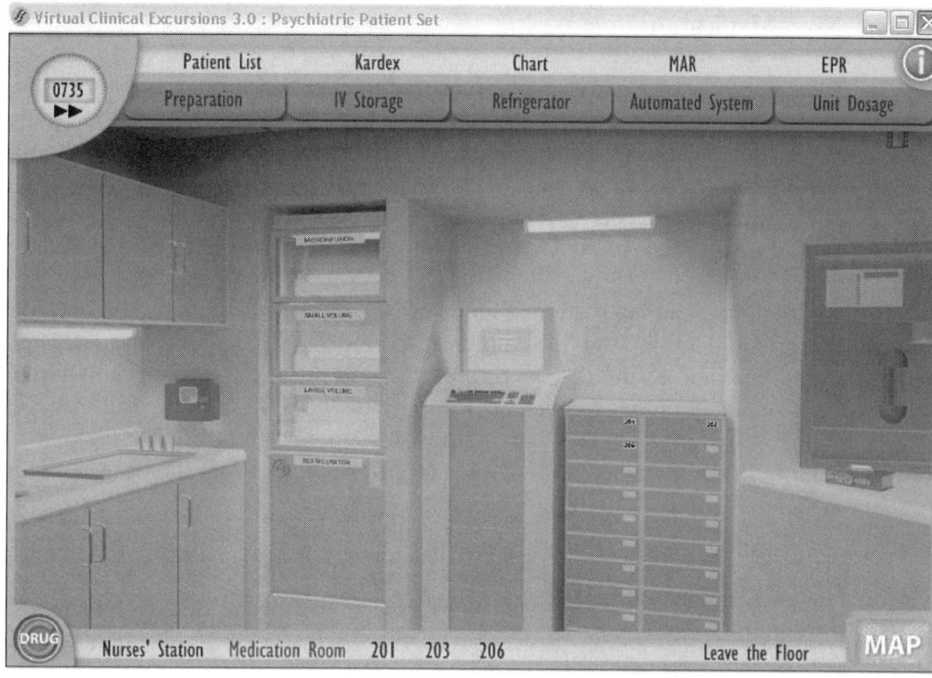

In the Medication Room you have access to the following (from left to right):

- A preparation area is located on the counter under the cabinets. To begin the medication preparation process, click on the tray on the counter or click on the **Preparation** icon at the top of the screen. The next screen leads you through a specific sequence (called the Preparation Wizard) to prepare medications one at a time for administration to a patient. However, no medication has been selected at this time. We will do this while working with a patient in *A Detailed Tour*. To exit this screen, click on **View Medication Room**.

- To the right of the cabinets (and above the refrigerator), IV storage bins are provided. Click on the bins themselves or on the **IV Storage** icon at the top of the screen. The bins are labeled **Microinfusion**, **Small Volume**, and **Large Volume**. Click on an individual bin to see a list of its contents. If you needed to prepare an IV medication at this time, you could click on the medication and its label would appear to the right under the patient's name. (*Note:* You can **Open** and **Close** any medication label by clicking the appropriate icon.) Next, you would click **Put Medication on Tray**. If you ever change your mind or decide that you have put the incorrect medication on the tray, you can reverse your actions by highlighting the medication on the tray and then clicking **Put Medication in Bin**. Click **Close Bin** in the right bottom corner to exit. **View Medication Room** brings you back to a full view of the entire room.

- A refrigerator is located under the IV storage bins to hold any medications that must be stored below room temperature. Click on the refrigerator door or on the **Refrigerator** icon at the top of the screen. Then click on the close-up view of the door to access the medications. When you are finished, click **Close Door** and then **View Medication Room**.

- To prepare controlled substances, click the **Automated System** icon at the top of the screen or click the computer monitor located to the right of the IV storage bins. A login screen will appear; your name and password are automatically filled in. Click **Login**. Select the patient for whom you wish to access medications; then select the correct medication drawer to open (they are stored alphabetically). Click **Open Drawer**, highlight the proper medication, and choose **Put Medication on Tray**. When you are finished, click **Close Drawer** and then **View Medication Room**.

- Next to the Automated System is a set of drawers identified by patient room number. To access these, click on the drawers or on the **Unit Dosage** icon at the top of the screen. This provides a close-up view of the drawers. To open a drawer, click on the room number of the patient you are working with. Next, click on the medication you would like to prepare for the patient, and a label will appear, listing the medication strength, units, and dosage per unit. To exit, click **Close Drawer**; then click **View Medication Room**.

At any time, you can learn about a medication you wish to prepare for a patient by clicking on the **Drug** icon in the bottom left corner of the medication room screen or by clicking the **Drug Guide** book on the counter to the right of the unit dosage drawers. The **Drug Guide** provides information about the medications commonly included in nursing drug handbooks. Nutritional supplements and maintenance intravenous fluid preparations are not included. Highlight a medication in the alphabetical list; relevant information about the drug will appear in the screen below. To exit, click **Return to Medication Room**.

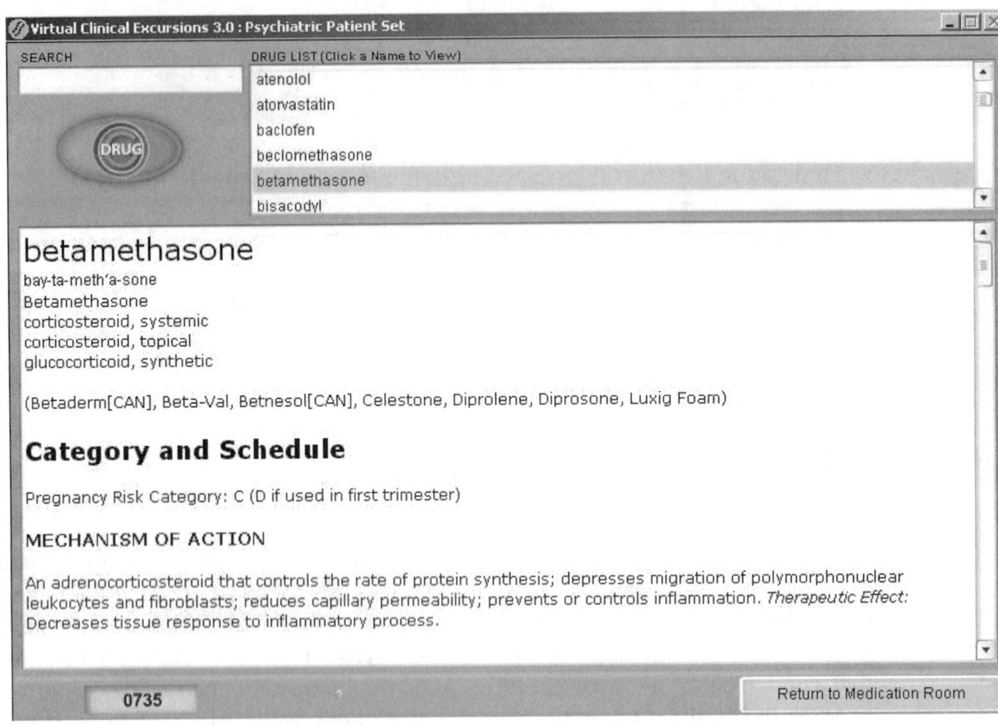

To access the MAR to review the medications ordered for a patient, click on the **MAR** icon located in the tool bar at the top of your screen and then click on the correct tab for your patient's room number. You may also click the **Review MAR** icon in the tool bar at the bottom of your screen from inside each medication storage area.

After you have chosen and prepared medications, go to the patient's room to administer them by clicking on the room number in the bottom tool bar. Inside the patient's room, click **Patient Care** and then **Medication Administration** and follow the proper administration sequence.

PRECEPTOR'S EVALUATIONS

When you have finished a session, click on **Leave the Floor** to go to the Floor Menu. At this point, you can click on the top icon (**Look at Your Preceptor's Evaluation**) to receive a scorecard that provides feedback on the work you completed during patient care.

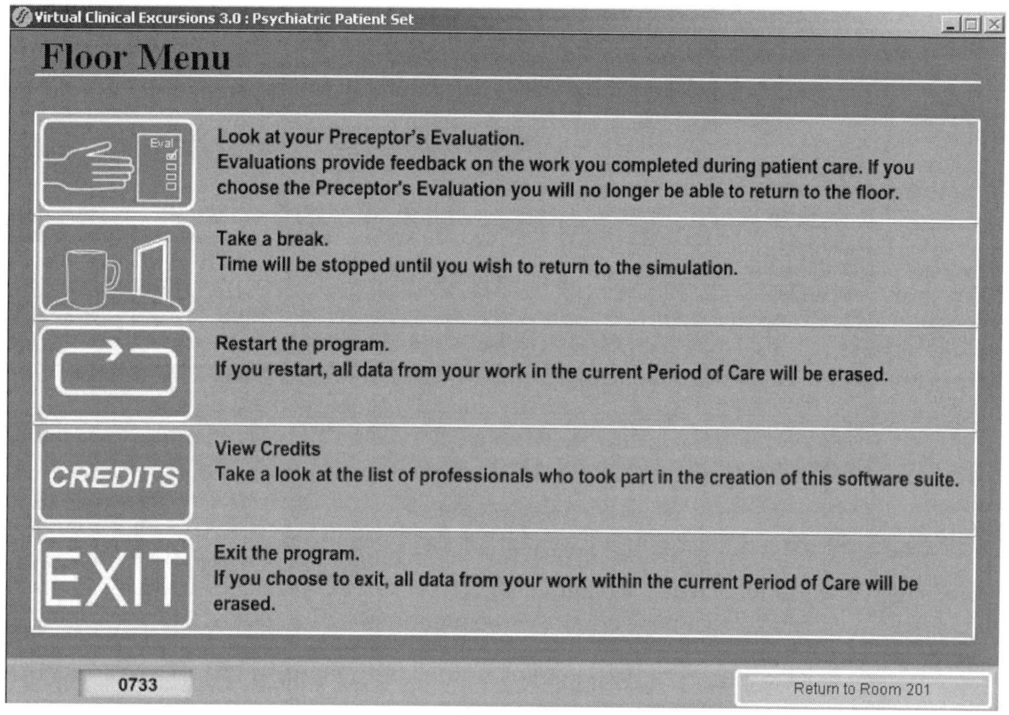

Evaluations are available for each patient you selected when you signed in for the current period of care. Click on the **Medication Scorecard** icon to see an example.

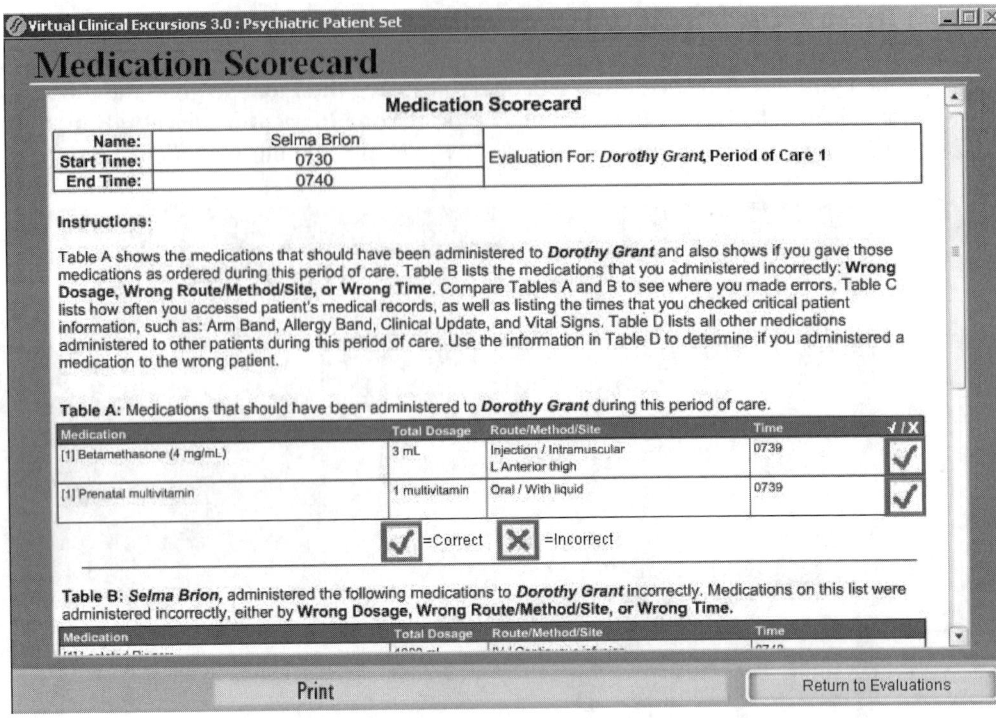

The scorecard compares the medications you administered to a patient during a period of care with what should have been administered. Table A lists the correct medications. Table B lists any medications that were administered incorrectly.

Remember, not every medication listed on the MAR should necessarily be given. For example, a patient might have an allergy to a drug that was ordered, or a medication might have been improperly transcribed to the MAR. Predetermined medication "errors" embedded within the program challenge you to exercise critical thinking skills and professional judgment when deciding to administer a medication, just as you would in a real hospital. Use all your available resources, such as the patient's chart and the MAR, to make your decision.

Table C lists the resources that were available to assist you in medication administration. It also documents whether and when you accessed these resources. For example, did you check the patient armband or perform a check of vital signs? If so, when?

You can click **Print** to get a copy of this report if needed. When you have finished reviewing the scorecard, click **Return to Evaluations** and then **Return to Menu**.

FLOOR MAP

To get a general sense of your location within the hospital, you can click on the **Map** icon found in the lower right corner of most of the screens in the *Virtual Clinical Excursions—Psychiatric* program. (*Note:* If you are following this quick tour step by step, you will need to **Restart the Program** from the Floor Menu, sign in again, and go to the Nurses' Station to access the map.) When you click the **Map** icon, a floor map appears, showing the layout of the floor you are currently on, as well as a directory of the patients and services on that floor. As you move your cursor over the directory list, the location of each room is highlighted on the map (and vice versa). The floor map can be accessed from the Nurses' Station, Medication Room, and each patient's room.

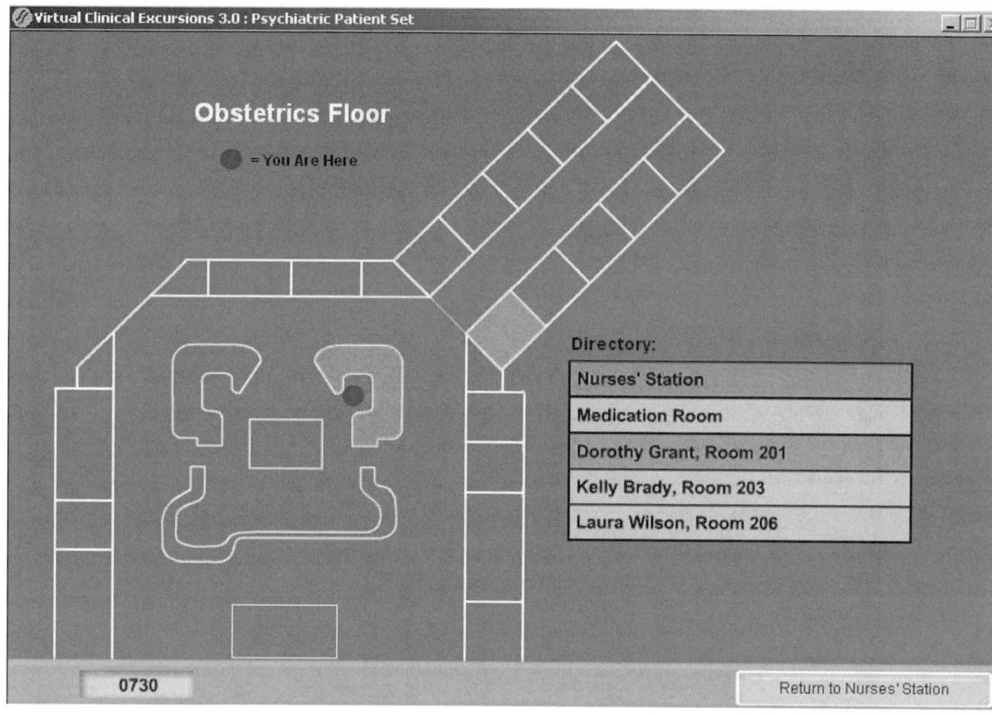

A DETAILED TOUR

If you wish to more thoroughly understand the capabilities of *Virtual Clinical Excursions—Psychiatric*, take a detailed tour by completing the following section. During this tour, we will work with a specific patient to introduce you to all the different components and learning opportunities available within the software.

■ WORKING WITH A PATIENT

Sign in and select the Obstetrics Floor for Period of Care 1 (0730-0815). From the Patient List, select Dorothy Grant in Room 201; however, do not go to the Nurses' Station yet.

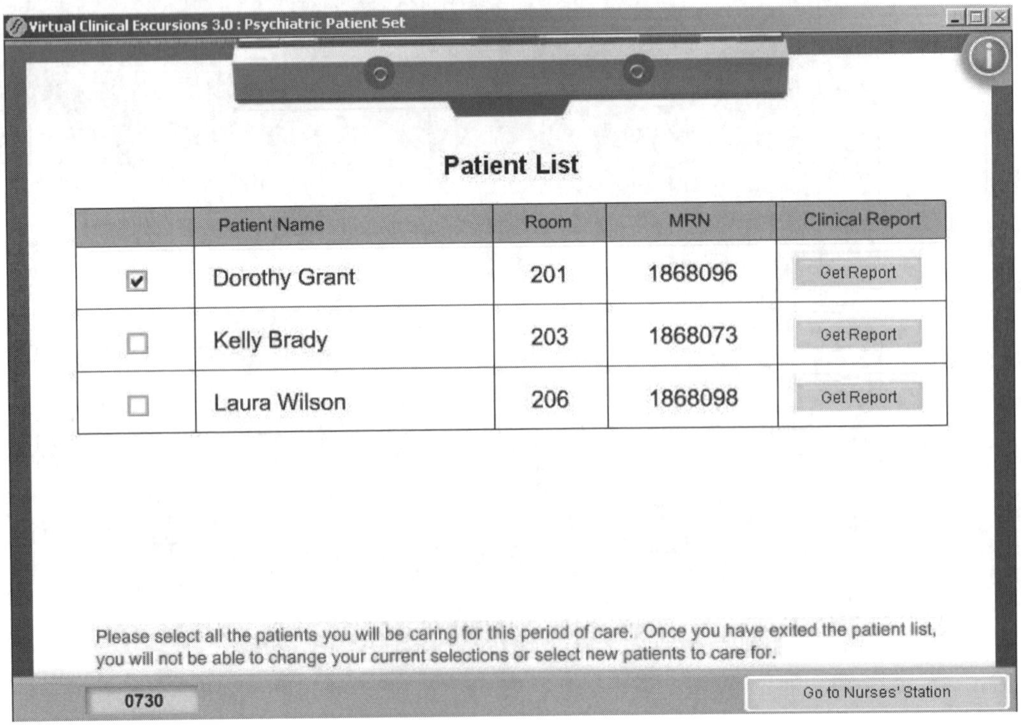

■ REPORT

In hospitals, when one shift ends and another begins, the outgoing nurse who attended a patient will give a verbal and sometimes a written summary of that patient's condition to the incoming nurse who will assume care for the patient. This summary is called a report and is an important source of data to provide an overview of a patient. Your first task is to get the clinical report on Dorothy Grant. To do this, click **Get Report** in the far right column in this patient's row. From a brief review of this summary, identify the problems and areas of concern that you will need to address for this patient.

When you have finished noting any areas of concern, click on **Go to Nurses' Station**.

CHARTS

You can access Dorothy Grant's chart from the Nurses' Station or from the patient's room (201). From the Nurses' Station, click on the chart rack or on the **Chart** icon in the tool bar at the top of your screen. Next, click on the chart labeled **201** to open the medical record for Dorothy Grant. Click on the **Emergency Department** tab to view a record of why this patient was admitted.

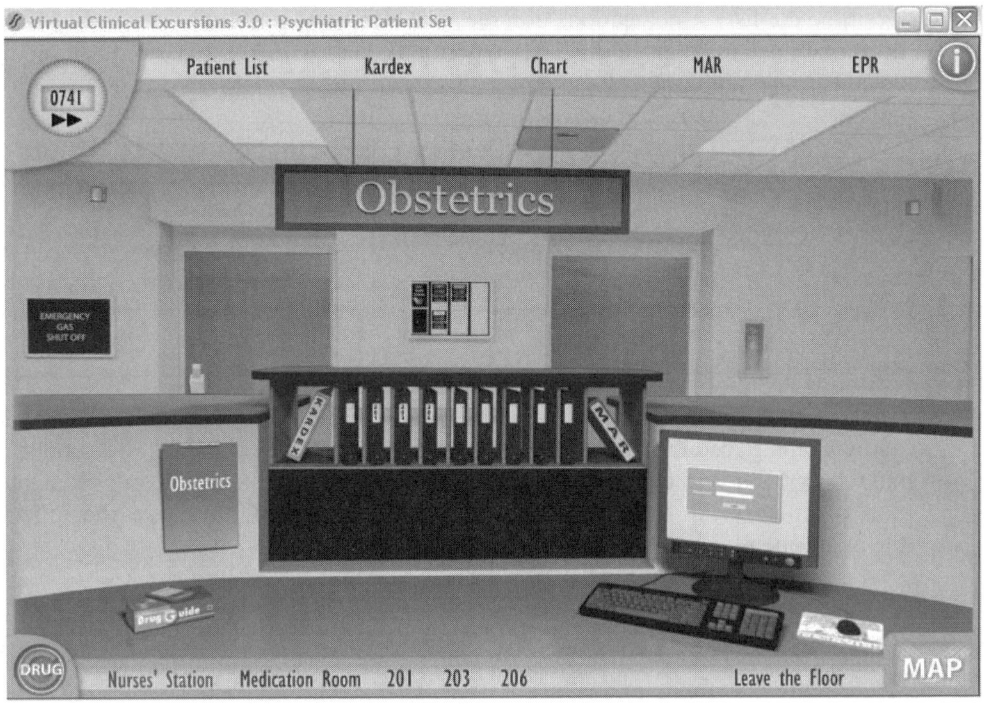

How many days has Dorothy Grant been in the hospital?

What tests were done upon her arrival in the Emergency Department and why?

What was her reason for admission?

You should also click on **Surgical Reports** to learn what procedures were performed and when. Finally, review the **Nursing Admission** and **History and Physical** to learn about the health history of this patient. When you are done reviewing the chart, click **Return to Nurses' Station**.

■ MEDICATIONS

Open the Medication Administration Record (MAR) by clicking on the **MAR** icon in the tool bar at the top of your screen. *Remember:* The MAR automatically opens to the first occupied room number on the floor—which is not necessarily your patient's room number! Since you need to access Dorothy Grant's MAR, click on tab **201** (her room number). Always make sure you are giving the *Right Drug to the Right Patient!*

Examine the list of medications ordered for Dorothy Grant. In the table below, list the medications that need to be given during this period of care (0730-0815). For each medication, note the dosage, route, and time to be given.

Time	Medication	Dosage	Route

Click on **Return to Nurses' Station**. Next, click on **201** on the bottom tool bar and then verify that you are indeed in Dorothy Grant's room. Select **Clinical Alerts** (the icon to the right of Initial Observations) to check for any emerging data that might affect your medication administration priorities. Next, go to the patient's chart (click on the **Chart** icon; then click on **201**). When the chart opens, select the **Physician's Orders** tab.

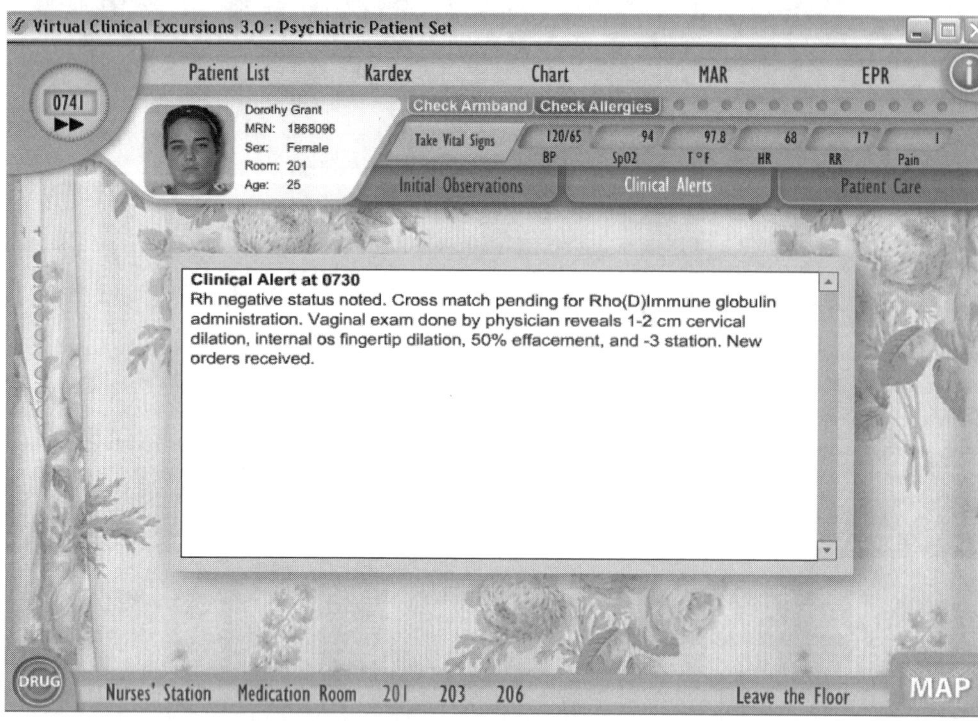

Review the orders. Have any new medications been ordered? Return to the MAR (click **Return to Room 201**; then click **MAR**). Verify that the new medications have been correctly transcribed to the MAR. Mistakes are sometimes made in the transcription process in the hospital setting, and it is sound practice to double-check any new order.

Are there any patient assessments you will need to perform before administering these medications? If so, return to Room 201 and click on **Patient Care** and then **Physical Assessment** to complete those assessments before proceeding.

Now click on the **Medication Room** icon in the tool bar at the bottom of your screen to locate and prepare the medications for Dorothy Grant.

In the Medication Room, you must access the medications for Dorothy Grant from the specific dispensing system in which each medication is stored. Locate each medication that needs to be given in this time period and click on **Put Medication on Tray** as appropriate. (*Hint:* Look in **Unit Dosage** drawer first.) When you are finished, click on **Close Drawer** and then on **View Medication Room**. Now click on the medication tray on the counter on the left side of the medication room screen to begin preparing the medications you have selected. (*Remember:* You can also click **Preparation** in the tool bar at the top of the screen.)

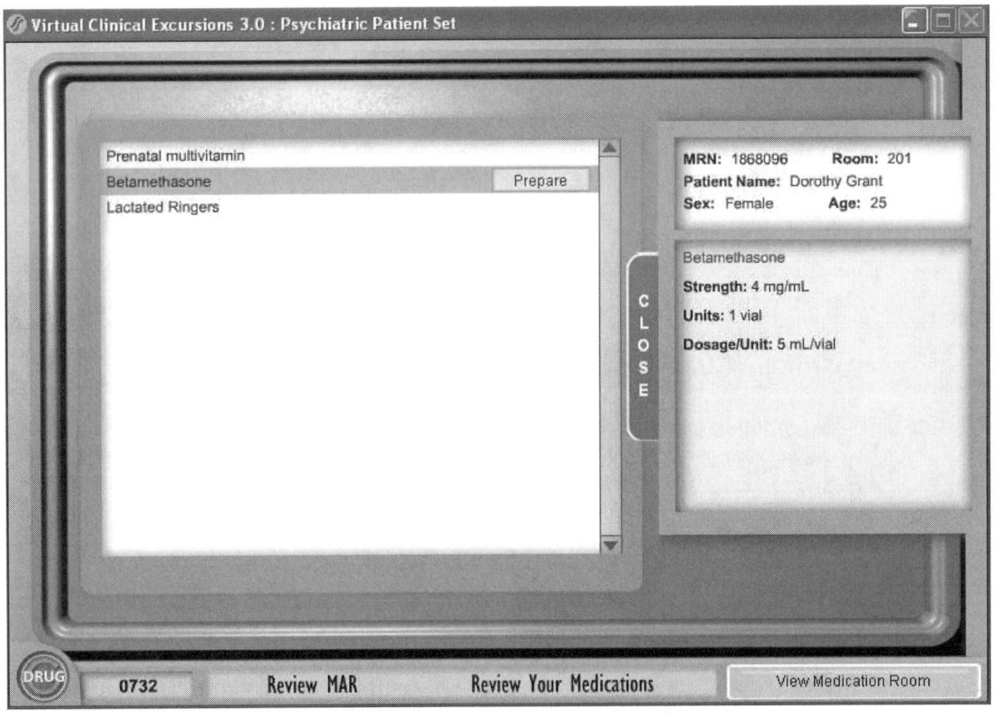

In the preparation area, you should see a list of the medications you put on the tray in the previous steps. Click on the first medication and then click **Prepare**. Follow the onscreen instructions of the Preparation Wizard, providing any data requested. As an example, let's follow the preparation process for betamethasone, one of the medications due to be administered to Dorothy Grant during this period of care. To begin, click to select **Betamethasone**; then click **Prepare**. Now work through the Preparation Wizard sequence as detailed below:

Amount of medication in the ampule: Betamethasone 5 mL.
Enter the amount of medication you will draw up into a syringe: **3 mL**.
Click **Next**.
Select the patient to receive the medication: **Room 201, Dorothy Grant**.
Click **Finish**.
Click **Return to Medication Room**.

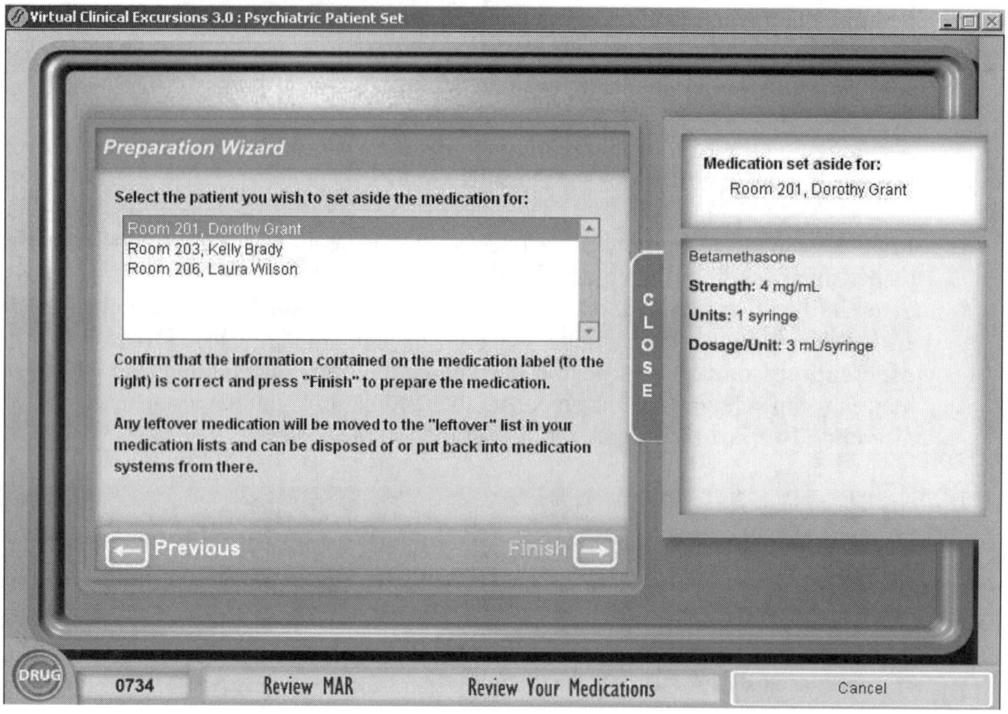

Follow this same basic process for the other medications due to be administered to Dorothy Grant during this period of care. (*Hint:* Look in **IV Storage** and **Automated System**.)

PREPARATION WIZARD EXCEPTIONS

- Some medications in *Virtual Clinical Excursions—Psychiatric* are prepared by the pharmacy (e.g., IV antibiotics) and taken to the patient room as a whole. This is common practice in most hospitals.
- Blood products are not administered by students through the *Virtual Clinical Excursions—Psychiatric* simulations since blood administration follows specific protocols not covered in this program.
- The *Virtual Clinical Excursions—Psychiatric* simulations do not allow for mixing more than one type of medication, such as regular and Lente insulins, in the same syringe. In the clinical setting, when multiple types of insulin are ordered for a patient, the regular insulin is drawn up first, followed by the longer-acting insulin. Insulin is always administered in a special unit-marked syringe.

Now return to Room 201 (click on **201** on the bottom tool bar) to administer Dorothy Grant's medications.

At any time during the medication administration process, you can perform a further review of systems, take vital signs, check information contained within the chart, or verify patient identity and allergies. Inside Dorothy Grant's room, click **Take Vital Signs**. (*Note:* These findings change over time to reflect the temporal changes you would find in a patient similar to Dorothy Grant.)

When you have gathered all the data you need, click on **Patient Care** and then select **Medication Administration**. Any medications you prepared in the previous steps should be listed on the left side of your screen. Let's continue the administration process with the betamethasone ordered for Dorothy Grant. Click to highlight **Betamethasone** in the list of medications. Next, click on the down arrow to the right of **Select** and choose **Administer** from the drop-down menu. This will activate the Administration Wizard. Complete the Wizard sequence as follows:

- Route: **Injection**
- Method: **Intramuscular**
- Site: **Any** (choose one)
- Click **Administer to Patient** arrow.
- Would you like to document this administration in the MAR? **Yes**
- Click **Finish** arrow.

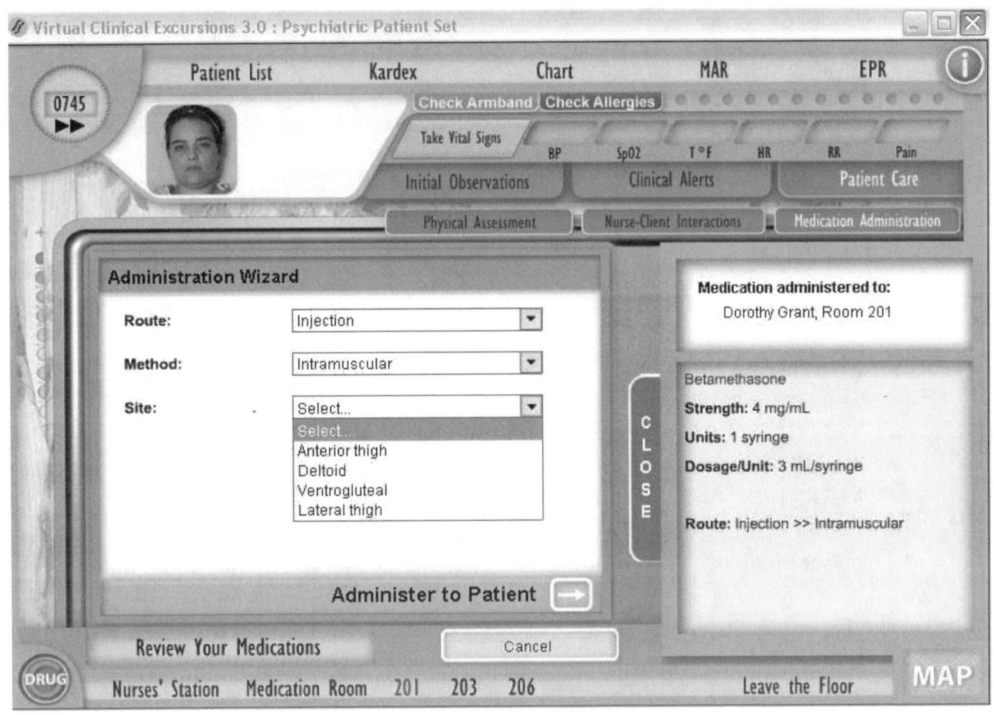

Your selections are recorded by a tracking system and evaluated on a Medication Scorecard stored under Preceptor's Evaluations. This scorecard can be viewed, printed, and given to your instructor. To access the Preceptor's Evaluations, click on **Leave the Floor**. When the Floor Menu appears, select **Look at Your Preceptor's Evaluation**. Then click on **Medication Scorecard** inside the box with Dorothy Grant's name (see example on the following page).

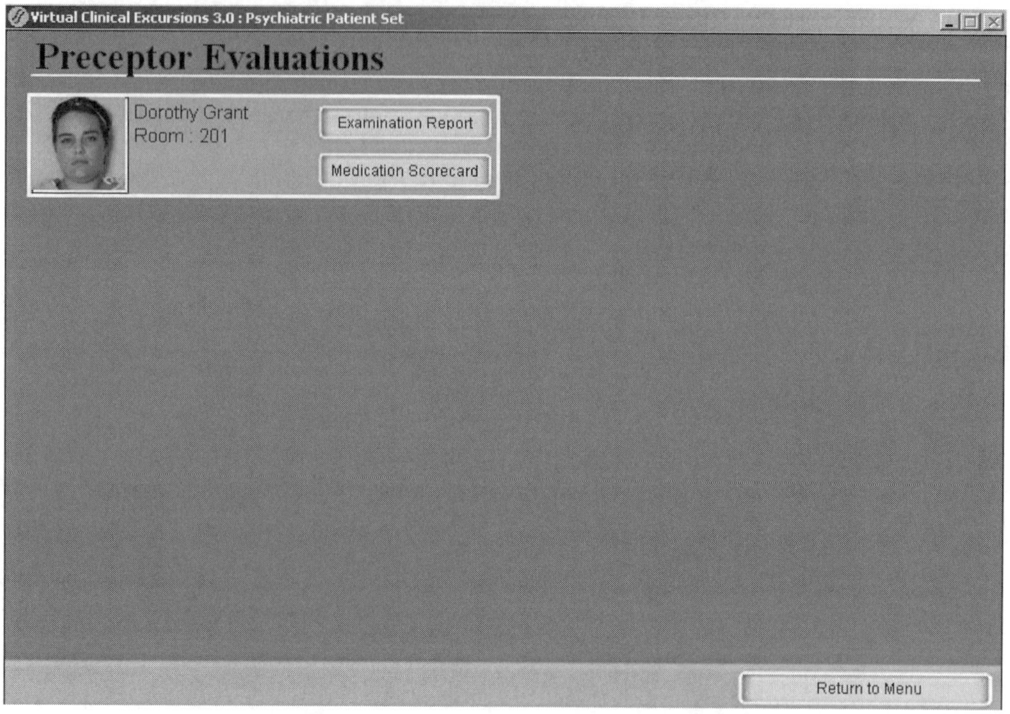

MEDICATION SCORECARD

- First, review Table A. Was betamethasone given correctly? Did you give the other medications as ordered?
- Table B shows you which (if any) medications you gave incorrectly.
- Table C addresses the resources used for Dorothy Grant. Did you access the patient's chart, MAR, EPR, or Kardex as needed to make safe medication administration decisions?
- Did you check the patient's armband to verify her identity? Did you check whether your patient had any known allergies to medications? Were vital signs taken?

When you have finished reviewing the scorecard, click **Return to Evaluations** and then **Return to Menu**.

VITAL SIGNS

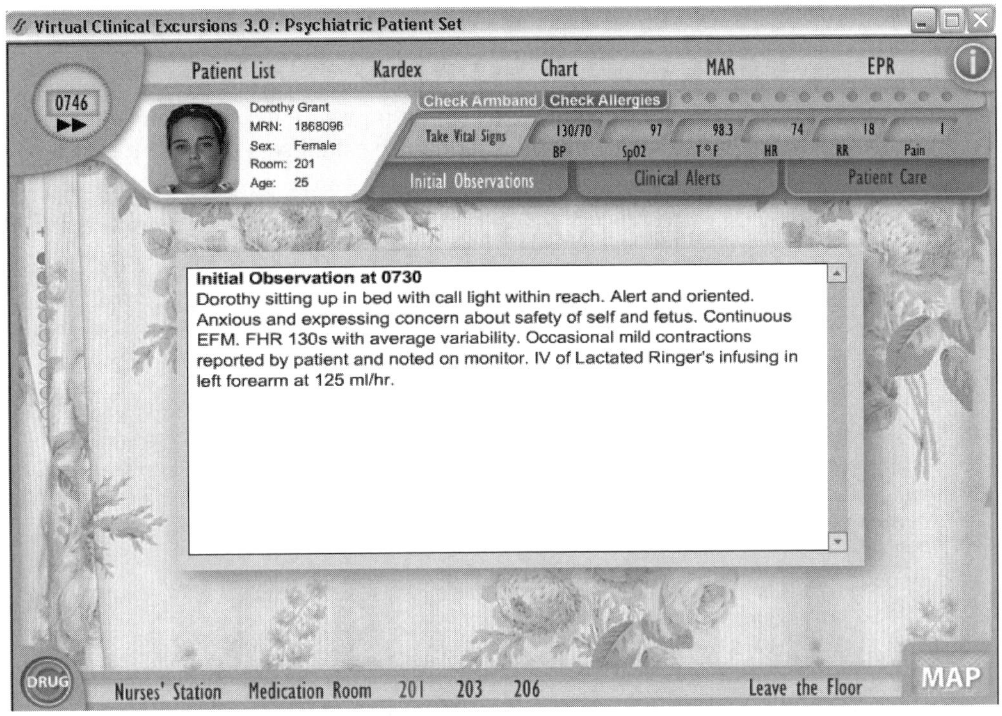

Vital signs, often considered the traditional "signs of life," include body temperature, heart rate, respiratory rate, blood pressure, oxygen saturation of the blood, and pain level.

Inside Dorothy Grant's room, click **Take Vital Signs**. (*Note:* If you are following this detailed tour step by step, you will need to **Restart the Program** from the Floor Menu, sign in again, and navigate to Room 201.) Collect vital signs for this patient and record them below. Note the time at which you collected each of these data. (*Remember:* You can take vital signs at any time. The data change over time to reflect the temporal changes you would find in a patient similar to Dorothy Grant.)

Vital Signs	Findings/Time
Blood pressure	
O_2 saturation	
Heart rate	
Respiratory rate	
Temperature	
Pain rating	

After you are done, click on the **EPR** icon located in the tool bar at the top of the screen. Your username and password are automatically provided. Click on **Login** to enter the EPR. To access Dorothy Grant's records, click on the down arrow next to Patient and choose her room number, **201**. Select **Vital Signs** as the category. Next, in the empty time column on the far right, record the vital signs data you just collected in Dorothy Grant's room. (*Note:* If you need help with this process, see page 16.) Now compare these findings with the data you collected earlier for this patient's vital signs. Use these earlier findings to establish a baseline for each of the vital signs.

a. Are any of the data you collected significantly different from the baseline for a particular vital sign?

   Circle One: Yes No

b. If "Yes," which data are different?

■ PHYSICAL ASSESSMENT

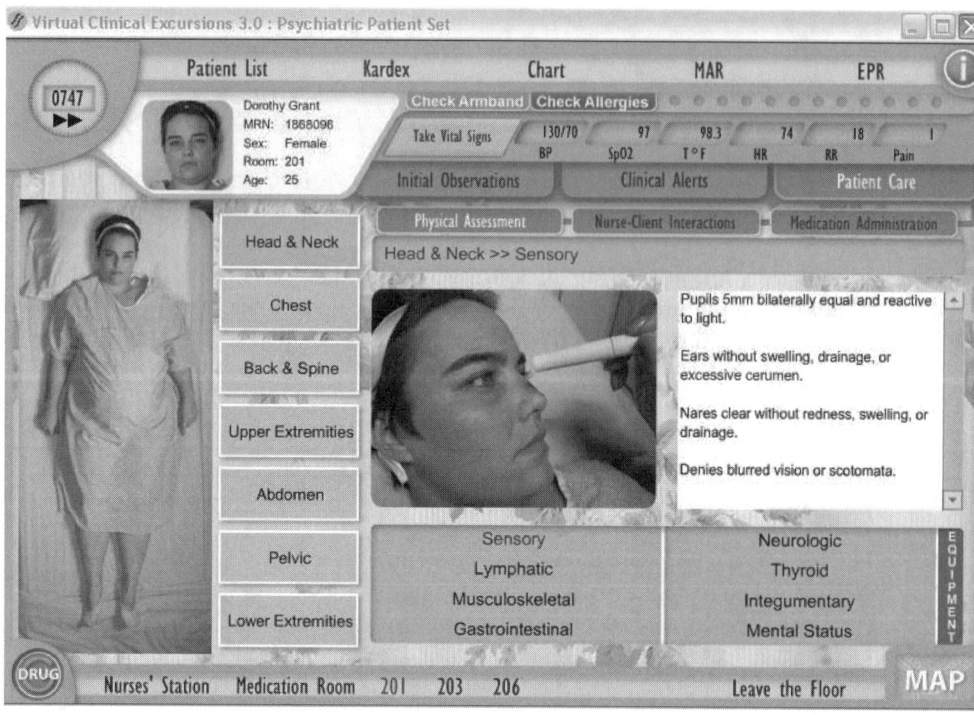

After you have finished examining the EPR for vital signs, click **Exit EPR** to return to Room 201. Click **Patient Care** and then **Physical Assessment**. Think about the information you received in the report at the beginning of this shift, as well as what you may have learned about this patient from the chart. Based on this, what area(s) of examination should you pay most attention to at this time? Is there any equipment you should be monitoring? Conduct a physical assessment of the body areas and systems that you consider priorities for Dorothy Grant. For example, select **Head & Neck**; then click on and assess **Sensory** and **Lymphatic**. Complete any other assessment(s) you think are necessary at this time. In the following table, record the data you collected during this examination.

Area of Examination	Findings
Head & Neck Sensory	
Head & Neck Lymphatic	

After you have finished collecting these data, return to the EPR. Compare the data that were already in the record with those you just collected.

a. Are any of the data you collected significantly different from the baselines for this patient?

   Circle One: Yes No

b. If "Yes," which data are different?

NURSE-CLIENT INTERACTIONS

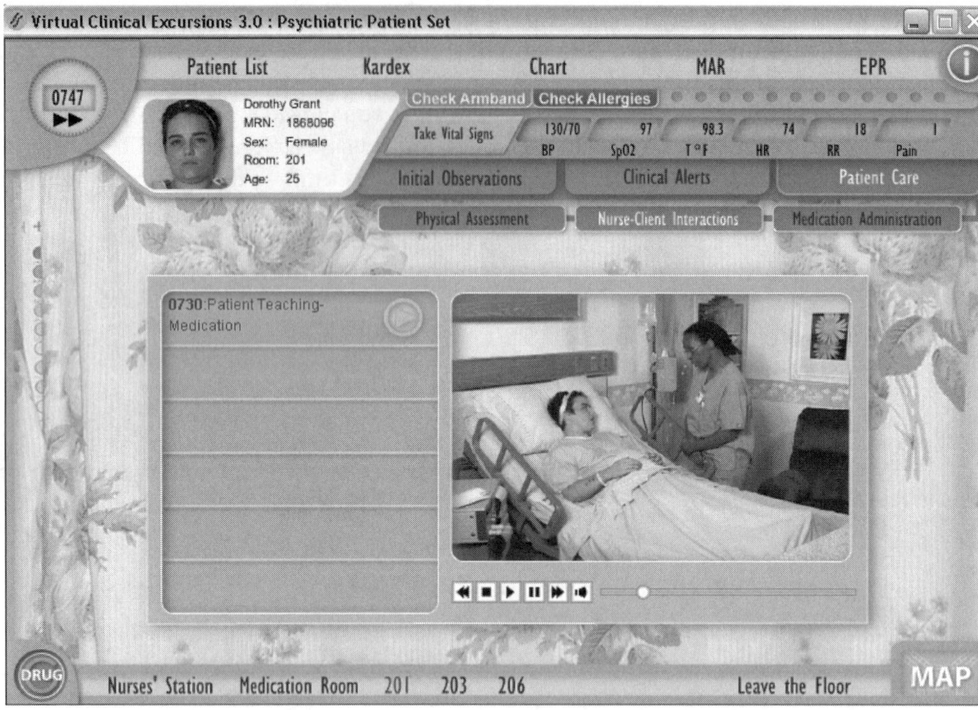

Click on **Patient Care** from inside Dorothy Grant's room (201). Now click on **Nurse-Client Interactions** to access a short video titled **Patient Teaching—Medication**, which is available for viewing at or after 0730 (based on the virtual clock in the upper left corner of your screen; see *Note* below). To begin the video, click on the white arrow next to its title. You will observe a nurse communicating with Dorothy Grant. There are many variations of nursing practice, some exemplifying "best" practice and some not. Note whether the nurse in this interaction displays professional behavior and compassionate care. Are her words congruent with what is going on with the patient? Does this interaction "feel right" to you? If not, how would you handle this situation differently? Explain.

Note: If the video you wish to view is not listed, this means you have not yet reached the correct virtual time to view that video. Check the virtual clock; you may return to access the video once its designated time has occurred—as long as you do so within the same period of care. Or you can click on the fast-forward icon within the virtual clock to advance the time by 2-minute intervals. You will then need to click again on **Patient Care** and **Nurse-Client Interactions** to refresh the screen.

At least one Nurse-Client Interactions video is available during each period of care. Viewing these videos can help you learn more about what is occurring with a patient at a certain time and also prompt you to discern between nurse communications that are ideal and those that need improvement. Compassionate care and the ability to communicate clearly are essential components of delivering quality nursing care, and it is during your clinical time that you will begin to refine these skills.

COLLECTING AND EVALUATING DATA

Each of the activities you perform in the Patient Care environment generates a significant amount of assessment data. Remember that after you collect data, you can record your findings in the EPR. You can also review the EPR, patient's chart, videos, and MAR at any time. You will get plenty of practice collecting and then evaluating data in context of the patient's course.

Now, here's an important question for you:

> Did the previous sequence of exercises provide the most efficient way to assess Dorothy Grant?

For example, you went to the patient's room to get vital signs, then back to the EPR to enter data and compare your findings with extant data. Next, you went back to the patient's room to do a physical examination, then again back to the EPR to enter and review data. If this back-and-forth process of data collection and recording seemed inefficient, remember the following:

- Plan all of your nursing activities to maximize efficiency, while at the same time optimizing the quality of patient care. (Think about what data you might need before performing certain tasks. For example, do you need to check a heart rate before administering a cardiac medication or check an IV site before starting an infusion?)
- You collect a tremendous amount of data when you work with a patient. Very few people can accurately remember all these data for more than a few minutes. Develop efficient assessment skills, and record data as soon as possible after collecting them.
- Assessment data are only the starting point for the nursing process.

Make a clear distinction between these first exercises and how you actually provide nursing care. These initial exercises were designed to involve you actively in the use of different software components. This workbook focuses on sensible practices for implementing the nursing process in ways that ensure the highest-quality care of patients.

Most important, remember that a human being changes through time, and that these changes include both the physical and psychosocial facets of a person as a living organism. Think about this for a moment. Some patients may change physically in a very short time (a patient with emerging myocardial infarction) or more slowly (a patient with a chronic illness). Patients' overall physical and psychosocial conditions may improve or deteriorate. They may have effective coping skills and familial support, or they may feel alone and full of despair. In fact, each individual is a complex mix of physical and psychosocial elements, and at least some of these elements usually change through time.

Thus it is crucial that you *DO NOT* think of the nursing process as a simple one-time, five-step procedure consisting of assessment, nursing diagnosis, planning, implementation, and evaluation. Rather, the nursing process should be utilized as a creative and systematic approach to delivering nursing care. Furthermore, because all living organisms are constantly changing, we must apply the nursing process over and over. Each time we follow the nursing process for an individual patient, we refine our understanding of that patient's physical and psychosocial conditions based on collection and analysis of many different types of data. *Virtual Clinical Excursions—Psychiatric* will help you develop both the creativity and the systematic approach needed to become a nurse who is equipped to deliver the highest-quality care to all patients.

REDUCING MEDICATION ERRORS

Earlier in this detailed tour, you learned the basic steps of medication preparation and administration. The following simulations will allow you to practice those skills further—with an increased emphasis on reducing medication errors by using the Medication Scorecard to evaluate your work.

Sign in to work on the Obstetrics Floor at Pacific View Regional Hospital for Period of Care 1. (*Note:* If you are already working with another patient or during another period of care, click on **Leave the Floor** and then **Restart the Program**; then sign in.)

From the Patient List, select Dorothy Grant. Then click on **Go to Nurses' Station**. Complete the following steps to prepare and administer medications to Dorothy Grant.

- Click on **Medication Room**.
- Click on **MAR** and then on tab **201** to determine prn medications that have been ordered for Dorothy Grant. (*Note:* You may click on **Review MAR** at any time to verify the correct medication orders. Always remember to check the patient name on the MAR to make sure you have the correct patient's record—you must click on the correct room number tab within the MAR.) Click on **Return to Medication Room** after reviewing the correct MAR.
- Click on **Unit Dosage** (or on the Unit Dosage cabinet); from the close-up view, click on drawer **201**.
- Select the medications you would like to administer. After each selection, click **Put Medication on Tray**. When you are finished selecting medications, click **Close Drawer** and then **View Medication Room**.
- Click on **Automated System** (or on the Automated System unit itself). Click **Login**.
- On the next screen, specify the correct patient and drawer location.
- Select the medication you would like to administer and click **Put Medication on Tray**. Repeat this process if you wish to administer other medications from the Automated System.
- When you are finished, click **Close Drawer** and **View Medication Room**.
- From the Medication Room, click **Preparation** (or on the preparation tray).
- From the list of medications on your tray, highlight the correct medication to administer and click **Prepare**.
- This activates the Preparation Wizard. Supply any requested information; then click **Next**.
- Now select the correct patient to receive this medication and click **Finish**.
- Repeat the previous three steps until all medications that you want to administer are prepared.
- You can click **Review Your Medications** and then **Return to Medication Room** when ready. Once you are back in the Medication Room, go directly to Dorothy Grant's room by clicking on **201** at the bottom of the screen.
- Inside the patient's room, administer the medication, utilizing the five rights of medication administration. After you have collected the appropriate assessment data and are ready for administration, click **Patient Care** and then **Medication Administration**. Verify that the correct patient and medication(s) appear in the left-hand window. Highlight the first medication you wish to administer; then click the down arrow next to Select. From the drop-down menu, select **Administer** and complete the Administration Wizard by providing any information requested. When the Wizard stops asking for information, click **Administer to Patient**. Specify **Yes** when asked whether this administration should be recorded in the MAR. Finally, click **Finish**.

■ SELF-EVALUATION

Now let's see how you did during your medication administration!

- Click on **Leave the Floor** at the bottom of your screen. From the Floor Menu, select **Look at Your Preceptor's Evaluation**. Then click on **Medication Scorecard**.

The following exercises will help you identify medication errors, investigate possible reasons for these errors, and reduce or prevent medication errors in the future.

1. Start by examining Table A. These are the medications you should have given to Dorothy Grant during this period of care. If each of the medications in Table A has a ✓ by it, then you made no errors. Congratulations!

If any medication has an X by it, then you made one or more medication errors.

Compare Tables A and B to determine which of the following types of errors you made: Wrong Dose, Wrong Route/Method/Site, or Wrong Time. Follow these steps:

a. Find medications in Table A that were given incorrectly.
b. Now see if those same medications are in Table B, which shows what you actually administered to Dorothy Grant.
c. Comparing Tables A and B, match the Strength, Dose, Route/Method/Site, and Time for each medication you administered incorrectly.
d. Then, using the form below, list the medications given incorrectly and mark the errors you made for each medication.

Medication	Strength	Dosage	Route	Method	Site	Time
	❑	❑	❑	❑	❑	❑
	❑	❑	❑	❑	❑	❑
	❑	❑	❑	❑	❑	❑
	❑	❑	❑	❑	❑	❑

2. To help you reduce future medication errors, consider the following list of possible reasons for errors.

   - Did not check drug against MAR for correct patient, correct date, correct time, correct drug, and correct dose.
   - Did not check drug dose against MAR three times.
   - Did not open the unit dose package in the patient's room.
   - Did not correctly identify the patient using two identifiers.
   - Did not administer the drug on time.
   - Did not verify patient allergies.
   - Did not check the patient's current condition or vital sign parameters.
   - Did not consider why the patient would be receiving this drug.
   - Did not question why the drug was in the patient's drawer.
   - Did not check the physician's order and/or check with the pharmacist when there was a question about the drug or dose.
   - Did not verify that no adverse effects had occurred from a previous dose.

Based on the list of possibilities you just reviewed, determine how you made each error and record the reason in the form below:

Medication	Reason for Error

3. Look again at Table B. Are there medications listed that are not in Table A? If so, you gave a medication to Dorothy Grant that she should not have received. Complete the following exercises to help you understand how such an error might have been made.

   a. Perhaps you gave a medication that was on Dorothy Grant's MAR for this period of care, without recognizing that a change had occurred in the patient's condition, which should have caused you to reconsider. Review patient records as necessary and complete the following form:

Medication	Possible Reasons Not to Give This Medication

   b. Another possibility is that you gave Dorothy Grant a medication that should have been given at a different time. Check her MAR and complete the form below to determine whether you made a Wrong Time error:

Medication	Given to Dorothy Grant at What Time	Should Have Been Given at What Time

c. Maybe you gave another patient's medication to Dorothy Grant. In this case, you made a Wrong Patient error. Check the MARs of other patients and use the form below to determine whether you made this type of error:

Medication	Given to Dorothy Grant	Should Have Been Given to

4. The Medication Scorecard provides some other interesting sources of information. For example, if there is a medication selected for Dorothy Grant but it was not given to her, there will be an X by that medication in Table A, but it will not appear in Table B. In that case, you might have given this medication to some other patient, which is another type of Wrong Patient error. To investigate further, look at Table D, which lists the medications you gave to other patients. See whether you can find any medications ordered for Dorothy Grant that were given to another patient by mistake. However, before you make any decisions, be sure to cross-check the MAR for other patients because the same medication may have been ordered for multiple patients. Use the following form to record your findings:

Medication	Should Have Been Given to Dorothy Grant	Given by Mistake to

5. Now take some time to review the medication exercises you just completed. Use the form below to create an overall analysis of what you have learned. Once again, record each of the medication errors you made, including the type of each error. Then, for each error you made, indicate specifically what you would do differently to prevent this type of error from occurring again.

Medication	Type of Error	Error Prevention Tactic

Submit this form to your instructor if required as a graded assignment, or simply use these exercises to improve your understanding of medication errors and how to reduce them.

Name: ______________________________ Date: ________________

The following icons are used throughout this workbook to help you quickly identify particular activities and assignments:

Indicates a reading assignment—tells you which textbook chapter(s) you should read before starting each lesson

Indicates a writing activity

Marks the beginning of an interactive CD-ROM activity—signals you to open or return to your *Virtual Clinical Excursions—Psychiatric* CD-ROM

Indicates additional CD-ROM instructions

Indicates questions and activities that require you to consult your textbook

Indicates the approximate time required to complete an exercise

LESSON 1

The Nursing Process

Reading Assignment: The Nursing Process (Chapter 3)

Client: Harry George, Medical-Surgical Floor, Room 401

Goal: To understand the role of the nurse in caring for a complex client using the nursing process.

Objectives:

- Define the six steps in the nursing process.
- Discuss the value of documentation.
- Describe critical thinking as part of the nursing process.
- Use the nursing process in caring for a complex client.
- Compare and contrast medical diagnoses with nursing diagnoses.
- Use assessment data to formulate a plan of care.
- Describe two types of formats for treatment planning.
- Discuss the psychosocial aspects of treatment planning.

Exercise 1

Clinical Preparation: Writing Activity

30 minutes

1. In caring for clients, the professional nurse uses a six-step nursing process. Match each numbered standard with its corresponding name below.

	Nursing Process Standard	Name
_____	Standard I	a. Implementation
_____	Standard II	b. Outcome Identification
_____	Standard III	c. Assessment
_____	Standard IV	d. Evaluation
_____	Standard V	e. Planning
_____	Standard VI	f. Nursing Diagnosis

2. Discuss the value of documentation and the nurse's responsibilities for accurate documentation, sometimes viewed as the seventh standard of care.

3. Critical thinking, an essential component in the nursing process, combines judgment, intuition, and expertise. The critical thinking skills listed below and on the next page are used in all phases of the nursing process. Define each listed skill.

Critical Thinking Skill	Definition
Observing	
Distinquishing	

Critical Thinking Skill	Definition
Validating	
Organizing	
Categorizing	

4. The psychiatric *assessment* includes the client's mental status and psychosocial components. Therefore it is important that the nurse understand the aspects of each component. Match each of the following specific aspects to its corresponding component of the psychiatric assessment.

	Specific Aspect	**Component of Psychiatric Assessment**
_____	Appearance and attitude	a. Mental status
_____	Behavior and activity	b. Psychosocial
_____	Stressors and coping skills	
_____	Relationships	
_____	Mood, affect, and speech	
_____	Occupation	
_____	Culture and spirituality	
_____	Perception and thoughts	
_____	Sensorium and cognition	

5. From data gathered in the assessment, the nurse makes a *nursing diagnosis*. How would you describe a nursing diagnosis?

6. Discuss the differences between the Diagnostic and Statistical Manual (DSM-IV-TR) and the North American Nursing Diagnosis Association (NANDA).

7. *Outcome* statements consist of specific, measureable indicators that are used by nurses to evaluate the results of their interventions. Explain why outcome statements are such an important part of the nursing process.

8. The *planning* phase of the nursing process consists of the total planning of the client's overall treatment to achieve quality outcomes in a _______________, _______________, and _______________ manner.

9. Nursing *interventions* are critical action components of the implementation phase. Which of the following statements regarding nursing interventions are true? Select all that apply.

_____ They consist of the management and treatment approaches to identified health problems.

_____ They are selected to achieve client outcomes and to prevent or reduce problems.

_____ They are written in vague, general terms for individualized interpretation.

_____ Each intervention is based on a sound rationale.

_____ They are also known as nursing orders or nursing prescriptions.

10. Describe the two steps that the nurse takes in the *evaluation* phase of the nursing process.

Evaluation: Two-Step Process

Exercise 2

CD-ROM Activity

30 minutes

- Sign in to work at Pacific View Regional Hospital on the Medical-Surgical Floor for Period of Care 3. (*Note:* If you are already in the virtual hospital from a previous exercise, click on **Leave the Floor** and then **Restart the Program** to get to the sign-in window.)
- Select Harry George in Room 401.
- Click on **Go to Nurses' Station**.
- Click on **Chart** and then on **401**.
- Click on **History and Physical** and read the report.
- Click on **Nursing Admission** and read the report.

1. In reviewing the assessment data from the mental status and the psychosocial components of the H&P and Nursing Admission, what data do you believe are most important for the nurse to make a nursing diagnosis?

- Next, click on **Mental Health** and review the Psychiatric/Mental Health Assessment.
- Then click on **Consultations** and review the Psychiatric Consult for additional assessment information.

2. What additional mental status and psychosocial data do these documents provide to add to what is already known about Harry George?

3. Harry George's medical diagnoses are listed below. For each medical diagnosis, identify some examples of potential nursing diagnoses that may apply.

Medical Diagnoses	Potential Nursing Diagnoses
Major depressive disorder	
Substance abuse	

4. Write a clear, specific, and measurable outcome statement related to the nursing problems of restlessness, agitation, and combativeness.

5. According to your textbook, there are two accepted formats used for treatment planning that could greatly assist the nurse to plan, measure, and monitor Harry George's care. The two formats are ____ and the ______________________________.

6. Nursing interventions almost always include health teaching. Match the following types of health education interventions to the specific health topics Harry George will need during hospitalization and after discharge.

	Type of Health Education Intervention	Specific Health Topic
_____	Increase awareness of issues related to health and illness	a. Developing healthy coping skills such as stress reduction, motivation and self-esteem, problem solving, and stress management
_____	Increase understanding of potential stressors, possible outcomes, and alternative coping responses	b. Learning how to become clean and sober, how to care for himself, how to manage pain and diabetes, and how smoking cessation can positively affect his health
_____	Increase knowledge of where and how to obtain resources	c. Finding housing, finding and keeping a job, and locating family members
_____	Increase actual abilities	d. Dealing with the loss of his family and job, homelessness, and pain

7. According to the Psychiatric Consult in his chart, there is a plan to help Harry George meet his goals while in the hospital and after discharge. Which of the following components are found in his Psychiatric Consult? Select all that apply.

_____ Initiate sertraline, an antidepressant medication.

_____ Encourage him to enter a comprehensive alcohol/drug treatment program.

_____ Begin intensive long-term psychotherapy.

_____ Provide vocational rehabilitation skill training.

_____ Ask his relatives to provide him with a place to stay.

8. Current trends in health care delivery systems have shifted from inpatient facilities to community- and home-based settings, providing further opportunities for the nurse to use the nursing process. What hospital-based resources does the nurse have available to help Harry George with his needs after discharge to the community?

9. Taking into consideration Harry George's history and current needs, discuss how a positive change in his living/social environment could affect his rehabilitation and recovery.

LESSON 2

Therapeutic Communication

Reading Assignment: Therapeutic Communication (Chapter 4)

Clients: Jacquline Catanazaro, Medical-Surgical Floor, Room 402
Kathryn Doyle, Skilled Nursing Floor, Room 503

Goal: To understand the importance of the therapeutic nurse-client relationship and be able to identify and use therapeutic communication techniques with clients.

Objectives:

- Understand the characteristics and goals of therapeutic communication.
- Identify the personal qualities of the nurse that are necessary to communicate effectively.
- Define and discuss the importance of genuineness, positive regard, and empathy in the therapeutic nurse-client relationship.
- Identify the verbal and nonverbal components of communication.
- Discuss common types of boundary issues and their importance to the nurse-client relationship.
- Identify transference and countertransference in the therapeutic nurse-client relationship.
- Describe the phases of a therapeutic nurse-client relationship.
- Observe and identify effective communication techniques used by the nurse in nurse-client interactions.

In this lesson you will learn the essential elements of therapeutic nurse-client communication. You will observe and interpret nurse-client interactions to identify therapeutic verbal and nonverbal techniques. Begin this activity by reviewing concepts in Chapter 4 in your textbook.

Exercise 1

Clinical Preparation: Writing Activity

30 minutes

1. Communication, a dynamic, two-way, circular process, is influenced by several factors. List these factors.

2. Discuss the verbal and nonverbal components of communication.

3. Therapeutic nurse-client communication is the psychiatric/mental health nurse's single most important tool. List the characteristics and goals of therapeutic communication.

Characteristics of Therapeutic Communication	Goals of Therapeutic Communication

4. List personal qualities the nurse must have in order to communicate therapeutically with clients.

5. Discuss the qualities of genuineness, positive regard, and empathy that a nurse must have in order to establish and maintain therapeutic communication.

6. Establishing and maintaining boundaries are always imporant considerations in the nurse-client relationship. Two common circumstances that can produce blurring of boundaries are

____ and

____

____.

7. Two obstacles that can occur in the nurse-client relationship and affect the nature of the communication are transference and countertransference. Match each of these terms to its definition.

	Term	Definition
_____	Countertransference	a. Unconscious response in which the client experiences feelings and attitudes toward the nurse that were originally associated with other significant figures in the client's life.
_____	Transference	b. Response by the nurse toward the client; involves the nurse's specific emotional response to the qualities of the client and is inappropriate to the content and context of the therapeutic relationship.

8. Nurse-client relationships have three main phases. Match each phase of the nurse-client relationship to its characteristics.

	Phase	Characteristics
_____	Orientation	a. Signifies a loss for both the client and nurse; goals and objectives are summarized; progress is reviewed; regression is possible.
_____	Working	b. Trust is established, relationship is defined, contracts are established, and confidentiality and termination are discussed.
_____	Termination	c. Involves maintenance, gathering more information, promotion of client's strengths; behavioral changes are facilitated; resistance is overcome; problems and goals are evaluated; practice and expression of alternative adaptive behaviors are promoted.

Exercise 2

CD-ROM Activity

30 minutes

- Sign in to work at Pacific View Regional Hospital on the Medical-Surgical Floor for Period of Care 1. (*Note:* If you are already in the virtual hospital from a previous exercise, click on **Leave the Floor** and then **Restart the Program** to get to the sign-in window.)
- Select Jacquline Catanazaro in Room 402.
- Click on **Go to Nurses' Station** and then on **402** at the bottom of the screen.
- Click on **Patient Care** and then on **Nurse-Client Interactions**.
- Select and view the video titled **0730: Intervention—Airway**. (*Note:* Check the virtual clock to see whether enough time has elapsed. You can use the fast-forward feature to advance the time by 2-minute intervals if the video is not yet available. Then click again on **Patient Care** and **Nurse-Client Interactions** to refresh the screen.)

1. As you observe the 0730 video, make note of the therapeutic verbal and nonverbal communication techniques the nurse uses. Record these in the first column below. Then, for each technique you identify, list specific examples of verbal and nonverbal communication used by the nurse that demonstrate the technique. (*Hint:* See Table 4-2 on page 64 in your textbook.)

	Therapeutic Communication Techniques Used by Nurse	Specific Examples of Nurse Communication
Verbal		
Nonverbal		

Now let's jump ahead in time to observe a later interaction between the nurse and this client.

- Click on **Leave the Floor** and then on **Restart the Program**.
- Sign in to work with Jacquline Catanazaro on the Medical-Surgical Floor for Period of Care 2.
- Click on **Go to Nurses' Station** and then on **402** at the bottom of the screen.
- Click on **Patient Care** and then on **Nurse-Client Interactions**.
- Select and view the video titled **1115: Assessment—Readiness to Learn**. (*Note:* Check the virtual clock to see whether enough time has elapsed. You can use the fast-forward feature to advance the time by 2-minute intervals if the video is not yet available. Then click again on **Patient Care** and **Nurse-Client Interactions** to refresh the screen.)

2. As you observe the 1115 video, make note of the therapeutic verbal and nonverbal communication techniques the nurse uses. Record these in the first column of the table below. Then, for each technique you identify, list specific examples of verbal and nonverbal communication used by the nurse that demonstrate the technique. (*Hint:* See Table 4-2 on page 64 in your textbook.)

	Therapeutic Communication Techniques Used by Nurse	Specific Examples of Nurse Communication
Verbal		
Nonverbal		

Next, let's look at an interaction between the nurse and a different client.

- Click on **Leave the Floor** and then on **Restart the Program**.
- Sign in to work with Kathryn Doyle on the Skilled Nursing Floor for Period of Care 1.
- Click on **Go to Nurses' Station** and then on **503** at the bottom of the screen.
- Click on **Patient Care** and then on **Nurse-Client Interactions**.
- Select and view the video titled **0730: Assessment—Biopsychosocial**. (*Note:* Check the virtual clock to see whether enough time has elapsed. You can use the fast-forward feature to advance the time by 2-minute intervals if the video is not yet available. Then click again on **Patient Care** and **Nurse-Client Interactions** to refresh the screen.)

3. As you observe the 0730 video, make note of the therapeutic verbal and nonverbal communication techniques the nurse uses. Record these in the first column below. Then, for each technique you identify, list specific examples of verbal and nonverbal communication used by the nurse that demonstrate each technique. (*Hint:* See Table 4-2 on page 64 in your textbook.)

	Therapeutic Communication Techniques Used by Nurse	Specific Examples of Nurse Communication
Verbal		
Nonverbal		

LESSON 3

Cultural, Ethnic, and Spiritual Considerations

Reading Assignment: Cultural, Ethnic, and Spiritual Considerations (Chapter 7)

Client: Carlos Reyes, Skilled Nursing Floor, Room 504

Goal: To understand cultural, ethnic, and spiritual aspects of psychiatric nursing care.

Objectives:

- Understand how culture helps define mental health and illness.
- Define culturally competent care.
- Identify practice difficulties and methods to work through these difficulties to provide culturally competent care.
- Define characteristics of low- and high-context societies and their relevance in cultural care.
- Understand the role culture and spirituality play in the diagnosis and treatment of mental illness.
- Describe the positive aspects of spirituality for the client with mental illness.
- Describe how the nurse works with a family member of a client who is identified as Hispanic.

Exercise 1

Clinical Preparation: Writing Activity

30 minutes

1. Discuss how the DSM-IV-TR addresses syndromes unique to various cultures and how culture and religious beliefs might influence a client's level of compliance with treatment.

2. Indicate whether each of the following statements regarding the influence culture has on mental health and illness is true or false.

_____ a. Each cultural group has cultural beliefs, values, and practices that guide its members in ways of thinking and acting.

_____ b. The framework that describes mental health and illness in the United States is based on Eastern thought.

_____ c. Cultural differences deem what behavior is considered normal and what behavior is considered aberrant.

_____ d. The influence of a culture is so pervasive that people may fail to recognize cultural aspects of life.

_____ e. Culture is irrelevant when it comes to treating symptoms of mental illness.

3. In providing care to culturally diverse populations, the nurse will encounter difficulties in practice and must be knowledgeable about methods to overcome these difficulties. Listed below are three cultural practice issues and their associated difficulties. Complete the table by listing examples of how the nurse might work through each issue.

Cultural Practice Issue	Difficulty	Examples of Ways to Work Through Area of Difficulty
Communication	Language, meaning of nonverbal communication	
Diagnosis	Use of culturally inappropriate psychometric diagnostic tools	
Pharmacodynamics	Genetic variations in drug metabolism found in people of all ethnicities	

4. The purpose of ______________________________ is to ensure that clients of all cultures are given every opportunity to receive information about treatment in ways that they understand, considering their education, acculturation, and language.

5. Many approaches to understanding culture can be found in other disciplines such as anthropology, sociology, and psychology. One sociology framework that describes communication and behavioral aspects of culture has defined two types of societies: low-context and high-context. In the table below, list characteristics of these two types of societies and give at least one example of each.

Society Type	Characteristics	Example
Low-context		
High-context		

6. Describe the family characteristics of the Hispanic culture.

7. In order to perform a cultural assessment on Carlos Reyes, the nurse must identify key questions to include. Review Chapter 7 in your textbook and place an X next to each question you think should be included in Carlos Reyes' assessment.

_____ How old are you?

_____ What is your primary language?

_____ Would you like an interpreter?

_____ Who do you live with?

_____ Are there special foods you like to eat?

_____ How is your illness viewed by your culture?

_____ How tall are you? What do you weigh?

_____ What do you do to get better when you are medically ill? Mentally ill?

8. Spirituality plays an important role in mental health and can be crucial to the lives of many clients with mental illness. Some of the common issues experienced by mentally ill clients are listed below. Match each of these issues with a positive aspect of spirituality that may help the client with the issue.

	Positive Aspects of Spirituality	**Common Issues Experienced by Mentally Ill Clients**
_____	Provides a sense of being loved and accepted for who they are	a. Having a devastating chronic illness
_____	Gives a powerful sense of hope	b. Experiencing rejection by family and friends
_____	Provides a solid foundation	c. Feelings of abandonment
_____	Maintains a sense of connection and belonging	d. Feelings of internal chaos

Exercise 2

CD-ROM Activity

30 minutes

- Sign in to work at Pacific View Regional Hospital on the Skilled Nursing Floor for Period of Care 2. (*Note:* If you are already in the virtual hospital from a previous exercise, click on **Leave the Floor** and then **Restart the Program** to get to the sign-in window.)
- Select Carlos Reyes in Room 504.
- Click on **Go to Nurses' Station**.
- Click on **Chart** and then on **504**.
- Review the **History and Physical** and **Nursing Admission** records.

1. According to the medical record, Carlos Reyes' cultural background is ________________,

   and his religion is ___________________.

2. What are some characteristics of this culture?

3. Discuss the cultural factors that are important in caring for Carlos Reyes.

- Click on **Return to Nurses' Station**.
- Click on **504** at the bottom of the screen.
- Click on **Patient Care** and then on **Nurse-Client Interactions**.
- To answer questions 4-8, you will need to select and view the video titles listed below. (*Note:* Check the virtual clock to see whether enough time has elapsed. You can use the fast-forward feature to advance the time by 2-minute intervals if the video is not yet available. Then click again on **Patient Care** and **Nurse-Client Interactions** to refresh the screen.)
    - **0740: Family Teaching—Medication**
    - **0745: Drowsiness—Contributing Factor**
    - **0750: Assessment—Level of Assistance**
- After viewing the above three videos, click on the **Drug** icon in the lower left corner of your screen. Use the Search box or the scroll bar to find information on oxazepam.

4. The two interventions the nurse used to answer the concerns of Carlos Reyes' son regarding his father's drowsiness were ____ and ____________________ the client's medications as a cause for drowsiness.

5. What other actions could the nurse have taken?

6. Explain the indication for oxazepam and the effect it has on brain function. Identify the side effect that was concerning Carlos Reyes' son.

7. What aspects of the mental status exam is the nurse attempting to assess?

8. What level of assistance will Carlos Reyes need in order to sit up and eat his breakfast? Discuss the role of his family at mealtime.

LESSON 4

Adult Development in Later Life

Reading Assignment: Growth and Development Across the Life Span (Chapter 5)

Client: Kathryn Doyle, Skilled Nursing Floor, Room 503

Goal: To understand, assess, and care for the older client.

Objectives:

- Identify symptoms of mental illness in older adults.
- Discuss theories of aging from a variety of perspectives.
- Understand necessary skills of the geropsychiatric nurse.
- Acknowledge biases in working with the older client.
- Provide a comprehensive assessment of the older client.
- Identify common responses older adults have in relation to the aging process.
- Plan and coordinate the care for a geriatric client.
- Know effective treatment strategies to use with geriatric clients and their families.
- Evaluate the care given to the geriatric client.

Exercise 1

Clinical Preparation: Writing Activity

15 minutes

1. Mental health in late life depends on a number of factors. What factors do you believe might affect the mental health of older adults?

2. Ageism is an important issue that defines how a nurse will care for an older client. Define ageism and discuss its implications for health care delivery.

3. Positive attitudes toward older clients and their care must be included in nursing education programs. Each of the educational components in the table below would be important to include in a nursing education program. In the right column of the table, give a rationale for including each topic in teaching.

Educational Component	Rationale
Psychosocial aging	
Attitudes about working with older adults	
Healthy aging	
Sensitivity to needs of older adults	

4. To properly care for older adults, the nurse needs to have specialized knowledge and skills. Using the areas listed below and on the next page, identify specific knowledge and skills the nurse needs to have in order to work effectively with older clients.

Area	Specific Knowledge and Skills
Assessment	
Community resources	
Family and/or caregivers	
Medication	

Area	Specific Knowledge and Skills
Treatment modalities	
Advocacy	

5. Discuss possible biases you may have in working with older adults.

Exercise 2

CD-ROM Activity

45 minutes

- Sign in to work at Pacific View Regional Hospital on the Skilled Nursing Floor for Period of Care 2. (*Note:* If you are already in the virtual hospital from a previous exercise, click on **Leave the Floor** and then **Restart the Program** to get to the sign-in window.)
- Select Kathryn Doyle in Room 503.
- Click on **Go to Nurses' Station**.
- Click on **Chart** and then on **503**.
- Click on and read the **History and Physical**.
- Click on **Consultations** and read the Psychiatric Clinical Nurse Specialist Consult.

1. The four Ds of a comprehensive geriatric assessment are delirium, dementia, depression, and delusions. According to the medical record, Kathryn Doyle has depression. Depression is often confused with dementia and is not always recognized. Therefore, the nurse needs to be familiar with the symptoms of depression in later life. What symptoms is Kathryn Doyle experiencing that are consistent with later-life depression?

2. Kathryn Doyle seems to be experiencing anxiety. Indicate whether each of the following statements regarding anxiety in the elderly is true or false.

_____ a. Comorbid anxiety and depression are common in older adults.

_____ b. All types of anxiety combined are more prevalent than depression in older adults.

_____ c. Untreated anxiety can contribute to sleep problems, cognitive impairments, and decreased quality of life.

_____ d. Anxiety does not affect the family.

_____ e. Antianxiety medications also decrease depression.

3. Besides interviewing the geriatric client and completing a mental status exam, there are other components of the geropsychiatric nursing assessment. For each component listed below, identify the key elements to be assessed. Then, in the far right column, list data specific to Kathryn Doyle based on your review of her chart.

Component	Key Elements	Assessment of Kathryn Doyle
Behavioral responses		
Functional abilities		
Physiological responses		
Social support		

- Click on **Return to Nurses' Station** and then on **503**.
- Click on **Patient Care** and then **Nurse-Client Interactions**.
- Select and view the video titled **1150: Depression—Cause, Treatment**. (*Note:* Check the virtual clock to see whether enough time has elapsed. You can use the fast-forward feature to advance the time by 2-minute intervals if the video is not yet available. Then click again on **Patient Care** and **Nurse-Client Interactions** to refresh the screen.)

4. Depression and sadness are sometimes viewed as a normal part of aging. Kathryn Doyle's response to life events that have occurred over the past 9 months has resulted in a disturbance in her mood. What life events have led to Kathryn's mood disturbance, and what have been her responses to these events?

- Click on **MAR** and then on tab **503**.
- Review Kathryn Doyle's medication list.

5. Does Kathryn Doyle have medication ordered to treat her depression? Discuss the role of medication to treat depression in the elderly.

6. Based on the nurse's assessment, Kathryn Doyle has other affective, somatic, stress, and behavioral responses common to the older adult. Complete the table below by outlining her specific issues associated with these common reactions.

Type of Response	Issues Involved with Kathryn Doyle's Response
Situational low self-esteem	
Imbalanced nutrition	
Relocation stress syndrome	
Social isolation	

→ Let's jump ahead in virtual time to observe a later interaction between the nurse and Kathryn Doyle.

- Click on **Return to Room 503**.
- Click on **Leave the Floor** and then on **Restart the Program**.
- Sign in to work with Kathryn Doyle again, this time for Period of Care 3.
- Click on **Go to Nurses' Station**.
- Click on **503** at the bottom of the screen.
- Click on **Patient Care** and then **Nurse-Client Interactions**.
- Select and view the video titled **1505: Assessment—Elder Abuse**. (*Note:* Check the virtual clock to see whether enough time has elapsed. You can use the fast-forward feature to advance the time by 2-minute intervals if the video is not yet available. Then click again on **Patient Care** and **Nurse-Client Interactions** to refresh the screen.)

7. Elder neglect and abuse have become more common in our society as older people no longer have the status and respect they once had through their extended families. Serving as the client's advocate, the nurse must be alert for signs of elder neglect, abuse, or exploitation. What are the signs that Kathryn Doyle is being neglected, exploited, or abused?

8. During the family conference the issue of theft will be addressed. Another concern that needs to be discussed is Kathryn Doyle continuing to live in her son's home post hip fracture. If this living arrangement is to be successful, the home environment must include several basic characteristics therapeutic for older clients. List the environmental elements that must be included in Kathryn's home.

9. Most elders (about 80%) are cared for in the home. What topics should the nurse include in family education and support sessions that would be critical to Kathryn Doyle's recovery and future?

10. Aftercare for older clients is often necessary for a successful treatment outcome. After discharge what agency support do you think Kathryn Doyle's son will need in the care of his mother in the home?

LESSON 5

Caring for a Client with an Anxiety Disorder

Reading Assignment: Anxiety and Anxiety Disorders (Chapter 9)
Psychopharmacology (Chapter 24)

Client: Dorothy Grant, Obstetrics Floor, Room 201

Goal: To care for a client on an obstetrics floor who is experiencing anxiety.

Objectives:

- Define anxiety and identify its essential characteristics.
- Understand levels of anxiety.
- Describe physiological responses to anxiety.
- Define cognitive, behavioral, and affective responses to anxiety.
- Identify stressors leading to a client's anxiety.
- Identify outcome statements for clients with generalized anxiety disorder (GAD) and post-traumatic stress disorder (PTSD).
- Identify effective medications prescribed for clients with anxiety.
- Discuss levels of anxiety as they relate to nursing interventions.
- Develop treatment interventions and outcomes for a client with anxiety.

Exercise 1

Clinical Preparation: Writing Activity

30 minutes

1. Anxiety is defined as a universal human experience that produces a nonspecific vague feeling of _______________ with no identifiable _______________, resulting from an _______________ threat to one's integrity. The function of anxiety is to warn the individual of impending _______________, _______________, or _______________.

2. Match each level of anxiety to its characteristics.

	Level	Characteristic
_____	Mild	a. The perceptual field narrows as the person focuses on the immediate concerns
_____	Moderate	b. Associated with dread and terror; the personality becomes disorganized
_____	Severe	c. Associated with the tension of daily life
_____	Panic	d. Significant reduction in the perceptual field as the person focuses on details and cannot think of anything else

3. Identify at least two physiological responses to anxiety in each of the systems listed below and on the next page.

System	Physiological Responses to Anxiety
Cardiovascular	
Respiratory	
Gastrointestinal	

System	Physiological Responses to Anxiety
Neuromuscular	
Genitourinary	
Integumentary	

4. Match each type of response to anxiety with its group of characteristics.

	Type of Response	Characteristics
_____	Behavioral	a. Decreased attention, forgetfulness, loss of objectiveness, poor concentration, impaired judgment, preoccupation, thought blocking, decreased productivity
_____	Cognitive	b. Uneasiness, nervousness, impatience, jumpiness, fear, fright
_____	Affective	c. Rapid speech, restlessness, pacing, fine hand tremor, muscle tension, hyperventilation

5. ______________________________ are the primary methods the ego uses in an attempt to control or manage anxiety in order to protect individuals from painful awareness of feelings and memories that can provoke overwhelming anxiety.

6. Generalized anxiety disorder (GAD) is characterized by which of the following? Select all that apply.

_____ Excessive anxiety and worry that occurs most days for at least 1 month

_____ Anxiety that involves concerns about a number of events and activities

_____ Difficulty in controlling worry

_____ Anxiety and worry that interfere with social and occupational functioning

_____ Anxiety or worry that occurs as a result of using substances

7. There are general nursing interventions useful in working with clients with anxiety symptoms, regardless of the diagnosis. List five of these nursing interventions.

8. For clients with moderate to severe anxiety, medication may be a necessary intervention. In the table below, list the positive aspects and cautions associated with the use of antidepressant and anxiolytic medications in clients with anxiety.

Medication Class	Positive Aspects	Cautions
Antidepressants		
Anxiolytics		

Exercise 2

CD-ROM Activity

30 minutes

- Sign in to work at Pacific View Regional Hospital on the Obstetrics Floor for Period of Care 1. (*Note:* If you are already in the virtual hospital from a previous exercise, click on **Leave the Floor** and then **Restart the Program** to get to the sign-in window.)
- Select Dorothy Grant in Room 201.
- Click on **Get Report**.

1. According to the change-of-shift report, what level of anxiety is Dorothy Grant experiencing?
   a. Mild
   b. Moderate
   c. Severe
   d. Panic

2. It is reported that Dorothy Grant's stated concerns of ________________________ and the ____________________________________ are causing her anxiety.

- Click on **Go to Nurses' Station**.
- Click on **201** at the bottom of the screen.
- Review the **Initial Observations** the nurse made at 0730.

3. How does the nurse's assessment of Dorothy Grant's anxiety level compare with the assessment described in the change-of-shift report?

- Now click on **Chart** and then on **201**.
- Access and read the **Nursing Admission** section.

4. What are the two stressors listed that contribute to Dorothy Grant's anxiety?

5. Dorothy Grant is experiencing traumatic injury by her husband. What are your thoughts and feelings about this event?

6. Based on your review of outcome statements for PTSD and GAD in your textbook (pages 187 and 189), choose the outcome statements that fit best for Dorothy Grant's treatment plan. Select all that apply.

    _____ Exhibit enhanced ability to problem-solve and make decisions

    _____ Understand that medication only masks symptoms of increased anxiety

    _____ Demonstrate effective coping skills

    _____ Demonstrate concern for personal safety by starting to verbalize worries

    _____ Always uses own resources when a crisis occurs

7. You have assessed Dorothy Grant's level of anxiety to be moderate in severity. Develop nursing interventions based on the following aspects of treatment.

Aspects	Nursing Interventions
Recognition	
Insight	
Education	
Coping	

→ • Click on **Return to Room 201**.
• Now click on **MAR** and review Dorothy Grant's medications.
• Check to see whether there are any medications ordered for Dorothy Grant's anxiety.

8. What classification of medications would normally be ordered for a client with moderate to severe anxiety? Select all that apply.

_____ Stimulants

_____ Antidepressants

_____ Antipsychotics

_____ Antianxiety agents

_____ Mood stabilizers

9. In deciding whether to order medication to treat Dorothy Grant's anxiety, what are the key considerations?

LESSON 6

Caring for a Client with a Mood Disorder

Reading Assignment: Mood Disorder and Adjustment Disorders (Chapter 11)

Client: Kelly Brady, Obstetrics Floor, Room 203

Goal: To care for a client experiencing a medical health crisis who also has symptoms of depression.

Objectives:

- Understand lifetime prevalence of depression.
- Describe common risk factors and precipitating stressors in depression.
- Identify symptoms associated with depression.
- Discuss safety as it relates to the treatment of a client with depression.
- Assess a client who is experiencing depression.
- Develop a treatment plan for a client with depression.
- Understand the relationship between depression and pregnancy.
- Describe effective treatments including pharmacological treatment for depressed clients.
- Identify realistic discharge criteria for a client with depression.

Exercise 1

Clinical Preparation: Writing Activity

30 minutes

1. Mood disorders, particularly depression, are common. Which of the following statements about depression are true? Select all that apply.

   _____ Ethnicity and culture influence the expression of depressive symptoms.

   _____ Twice as many men as women develop depressive disorder.

   _____ Almost 20% of people in the general population will develop a mood disorder in their lifetime.

   _____ Depression is more prevalent in higher socioeconomic groups.

   _____ The average age for the onset of depression is in the mid-20s to 30s.

2. Depression may result from a complex interaction of causes and common risk factors. List potential causes and risk factors associated with depression.

3. For each type of symptom listed below and on the next page, provide examples seen in persons with major depression.

Type of Symptom	Examples
Affective/emotional	

Type of Symptom	Examples
Behavioral	
Cognitive	
Social	

4. When assessing a client with depression, the nurse must think about safety first. Explain the actions the nurse should take to make sure the client is safe.

5. People with depression have a genuine need to believe that things can get better. Select actions the nurse can take to instill hope in a client with depression. Select all that apply.

_____ Initially express hope to the client by discussing success in treating depression.

_____ Reinforce the fact that depression is a self-limiting disorder and that the future will be better.

_____ Explain to the client that depression is a chronic disease.

_____ Explain that untreated depression can lead to suicide.

_____ Inform the client that there are many very helpful medications and therapies available.

6. Based on what you know about the clinical course of depression, discuss measures you think would help prevent the recurrence of the disorder.

7. Evidence suggests that the psychotherapeutic intervention of cognitive therapy is an effective treatment for depression. Cognitive therapy addresses systematic errors in the client's

   ____________________. The goal of therapy is to identify underlying cognitive

   ____________________ and specific cognitive ____________________.

8. Successful behavior change is a powerful tool to counteract depression. List specific interventions the nurse can use with a depressed client to effect positive behavioral change, including possible activities that the client can do to accomplish this goal.

9. In clients with depression, which class of medication has proven the most effective with the least number of side effects?
   a. Selective serotonin reuptake inhibitors (SSRIs)
   b. Monoamine oxidase inhibitors (MAOIs)
   c. Tricyclic antidepressent drugs (TCAs)

10. Discuss the rationale for the nurse educating depressed clients on their illness and self-management strategies.

Exercise 2

CD-ROM Activity

30 minutes

- Sign in to work at Pacific View Regional Hospital on the Obstetrics Floor for Period of Care 1. (*Note:* If you are already in the virtual hospital from a previous exercise, click on **Leave the Floor** and then **Restart the Program** to get to the sign-in window.)
- Select Kelly Brady in Room 203.
- Click on **Go to Nurses' Station** and then on **203**.
- Review the **Initial Observations**.
- Click on **Patient Care** and then **Physical Assessment**.
- Click on **Head and Neck**.
- Click on **Mental Status**.

1. The two documented behavioral symptoms of Kelly Brady's depression are

   ________________ and ____.

2. Kelly Brady's depression follows the typical clinical course for depression. Based on what you have learned so far, which of the following statements apply to Kelly Brady's recurrence of depression? Select all that apply.

   _____ 50%-85% of clients with unipolar depression experience a subsequent episode.

   _____ Two-thirds of people with depression have a second occurrence within 10 years.

   _____ Recurrent episodes of depression tend to be increasingly intense.

   _____ There tend to be shorter time periods between recurrent episodes of depression.

   _____ The first episode of a mood disorder typically occurs in middle-aged adults.

- Click on **Chart** and then on **203**.
- Click on **History and Physical**.

3. The predisposing factor in Kelly Brady's family history related to depression is

   ____. In Kelly Brady's past medical history

   the key fact related to depression is ____

   ____.

Let's jump ahead to review a consultation that occurs later in the day.

- First, click on **Return to Room 203**.
- Next, click on **Leave the Floor** and then on **Restart the Program**.
- Sign in to work with Kelly Brady again, this time for Period of Care 3.
- Click on **Go to Nurses' Station**.
- Click on **Chart** and then on **203**. Select **Consultations**.
- Review the Psychiatric Consultation for Tuesday at 1500.

4. According to the Psychiatric Consult, Kelly Brady has major life events/precipitating stressors that contribute to her depression. What are the major life events and stressors that are contributing to Kelly Brady's depression?

5. List all the behavioral symptoms Kelly Brady is experiencing related to depression.

6. Develop a treatment plan to address Kelly Brady's depression by completing the intervention column of the table below and on the next page.

Area	Goal	Intervention
Environment/safety	To keep Kelly safe	
Cognitive	To move Kelly beyond her preoccupation to other aspects of her life	
Behavioral	To accomplish tasks and activities to counteract depression	

Area	Goal	Intervention
Social skills	To provide experiences to counteract depression and social isolation and build self-esteem	
Education	To educate Kelly about depression and the interventions and treatment that will be helpful	

7. Discuss how Kelly's pregnancy might be related to her depression.

8. Kelly's physician has recommended that she take paroxetine after the birth of her baby. Based on the medical records you have read, complete the medication information below.

   The trade name for paroxetine is ____________________, and the dose that was recommended is ______________. One clinical rationale for recommending paroxetine is that

   ____.

LESSON 7

Caring for a Client with Schizophrenia

Reading Assignment: Schizophrenia and Other Psychotic Disorders (Chapter 12)

Client: Jacquline Catanazaro, Medical-Surgical Floor, Room 402

Goal: To care for a client with chronic schizophrenia who is hospitalized for acute asthma.

Objectives:

- Define schizophrenia and discuss where it falls on the mental health continuum.
- Discuss the prevalence of schizophrenia.
- List the positive and negative symptoms of schizophrenia.
- Understand symptoms of schizophrenia and their impact on the cognitive, perceptual, emotional, behavioral, and socialization of the person.
- Identify predisposing factors and precipitating stressors of schizophrenia.
- Discuss the focus of treatment for each phase of schizophrenia.
- Identify communication techniques for clients exhibiting the positive symptoms of hallucinations and delusions.
- Describe the importance of education as part of the treatment for clients with schizophrenia and their families.
- Explain the importance of relapse prevention for clients with schizophrenia.
- Discuss medication as a treatment for clients diagnosed with schizophrenia.

Exercise 1

Clinical Preparation: Writing Activity

30 minutes

1. Schizophrenia is defined as a devastating and persistent neurobiological brain disease that profoundly and severely affects a person's ______________, ______________, ______________, ______________, and ability to perceive ______________ accurately.

2. The impact of schizophrenia on the individual and society is enormous. Read each statement below and indicate whether it is true or false.

_____ a. Men and women are equally represented in the population of individuals with schizophrenia.

_____ b. Of people diagnosed with schizophrenia, 100% have the disease for life.

_____ c. Most people who develop schizophrenia do not show symptoms until later adolescence.

_____ d. It is estimated that 5% of homeless people in the United States have schizophrenia.

_____ e. Addiction to alcohol occurs in approximately 30%-50% of individuals with schizophrenia.

_____ f. 50% of persons diagnosed with schizophrenia attempt suicide.

_____ g. 2% of the general U.S. population have been diagnosed with schizophrenia.

_____ h. Schizophrenia accounts for 20% of all hospital beds and 50% of all psychiatric beds in the U.S.

3. It is important to understand the positive and negative symptoms of schizophrenia. For each category listed below and on the next page, identify examples of associated positive and negative symptoms.

Category	Positive Symptoms	Negative Symptoms
Thinking		
Emotion		

Category	Positive Symptoms	Negative Symptoms
Speech		
Behavior		

4. Many stressors often precede a new episode or exacerbation of the symptoms of schizophrenia. Match each of the following specific stressors to its corresponding category.

	Common Relapse Stressor	Category of Stressor
_____	Low self-concept/self-confidence	a. Health
_____	Lack of social support	b. Environment
_____	Housing difficulties	c. Attitudes
_____	Aggressive/violent behavior	d. Behavior
_____	Lack of sleep	
_____	Poor medication management	
_____	Lack of transportation	
_____	Financial problems	
_____	Job pressures	
_____	Poor nutrition	
_____	Social isolation	
_____	Interpersonal difficulties	

5. In the assessment phase of the nursing process, the nurse conducts a mental status examination. For each category of the examination listed below, identify the most important questions to ask and observations to look for.

Mental Status Examination Category	Specific Questions/Observations
Disturbance in perception	
Thoughts	
Feelings	
Behavior	

6. As part of the implementation phase of the nursing process, discuss the importance of involving the client and the client's family in the treatment process.

7. Communicating with a client who has schizophrenia can be challenging. For each positive symptom listed below, identify three effective communication techniques the nurse can use with clients experiencing that symptom.

Positive Symptom	Communication Techniques
Hallucinations	
Delusions	

Exercise 2

CD-ROM Activity

45 minutes

- Sign in to work at Pacific View Regional Hospital on the Medical-Surgical Floor for Period of Care 3. (*Note:* If you are already in the virtual hospital from a previous exercise, click on **Leave the Floor** and then **Restart the Program** to get to the sign-in window.)
- Select Jacquline Catanazaro in Room 402.
- Click on **Go to Nurses' Station**.
- Click on **Chart** and then on **402**.
- Click on **Nurse's Notes**.
- Read the note written on admission on Monday at 1600.

1. Identify two pieces of information contained in the nurse's admission note that have implications for discharge planning. Select all that apply.

_____ Client has asthma.

_____ Sister is client's main support.

_____ Client has no transportation.

_____ Client has a history of stopping her psychiatric medication.

→ • Now read the **Nurse's Notes** dated Tuesday at 0400.

2. The statement made by the client that people are putting poison into her IV is an example of what type of delusion?
   a. Grandiose
   b. Persecutory
   c. Paranoid
   d. Fixed

→ • Now read the **Nurse's Notes** dated Wednesday at 0600.

3. The note describes symptoms of schizophrenia that have a direct relationship to Jacquline Catanazaro's asthma. Explain the relationship.

→ • Now click on the **Consultation** tab in the chart.
• Read the Psychiatric Consult.

4. The positive symptom of schizophrenia described in the report is ____________________, ____________________ and the negative symptoms described are ____ and ________________________________ ____________________.

5. The plan outlined in the Psychiatric Consult includes exercise and nutrition. Comment on the relevance of diet and exercise as part of the plan of care for Jacquline Catanazaro.

→ • Click on and review the **History and Physical** and **Nursing Admission** sections.

6. Relapse can be a devastating part of the disease of schizophrenia. For each category below and on the next page, list Jacquline Catanazaro's barriers to compliance that may result in future relapses.

Category	Barriers to Compliance
Health	
Thoughts	
Attitudes	

Category	Barriers to Compliance
Behavior	
Socialization	
Medication	

7. Education will be a critical component of Jacquline Catanazaro's treatment plan. Describe Jacquline's educational needs.

→
- Click on **Return to Nurses' Station** and then on **402**.
- Click on **Patient Care** and then **Nurse-Client Interactions**.
- Select and view the video titled **1500: Intervention—Patient Teaching**. (*Note:* Check the virtual clock to see whether enough time has elapsed. You can use the fast-forward feature to advance the time by 2-minute intervals if the video is not yet available. Then click again on **Patient Care** and **Nurse-Client Interactions** to refresh the screen.)
- Now click on **MAR** and then on tab **402**.
- Scroll down to locate the antipsychotic medication ordered.
- Click on **Return to Room 402**.
- Click on the **Drug** icon in the lower left corner of the screen. Find the entry for the medication you found in the MAR.

8. Based on your review of the Drug Guide, fill in the information specified below and on the next page for the antipsychotic medication ordered for Jacquline Catanazaro.

Name of medication

Indication

Mechanism of action

Side effects

Dosage

Nursing considerations

Client teaching

9. Consider the medication dosage Jacquline Catanazaro is receiving and the usual dosage listed in the Drug Guide. What might be the rationale for the current dosage the physician is giving to this client?

- Click on **Return to Room 402**.
- Click on **Patient Care** and then **Nurse-Client Interactions**.
- Select and view the video titled **1540: Discharge Planning**. (*Note:* Check the virtual clock to see whether enough time has elapsed. You can use the fast-forward feature to advance the time by 2-minute intervals if the video is not yet available. Then click again on **Patient Care** and **Nurse-Client Interactions** to refresh the screen.)

10. Discuss the importance of including Jacquline Catanazaro's sister in the discharge planning process.

LESSON 8

Caring for a Client with a Substance-Related Disorder

Reading Assignment: Substance-Related Disorders (Chapter 14)

Client: Laura Wilson, Obstetrics Floor, Room 206

Goal: To care for a client with acute medical needs who also has a diagnosis of polysubstance abuse.

Objectives:

- Discuss the prevalence of drug use in the United States.
- Differentiate between terms of abuse and dependence.
- Identify risks associated with drug use and pregnancy.
- Identify precipitating stressors, coping mechanisms, and resources of a client with polysubstance abuse.
- Discuss key assessment components of a client with polysubstance abuse.
- Identify key aspects of the treatment plan to include in teaching for clients with polysubstance abuse.
- Understand the importance of relapse prevention for a client with substance abuse.
- Describe critical elements of discharge planning for clients with substance abuse.

Exercise 1

Clinical Preparation: Writing Activity

15 minutes

1. Substance abuse disorders constitute a significant health problem in the United States. Read each statement below and indicate whether it is true or false.

    _____ a. In 2004, approximately 121 million Americans age 12 and over consumed alcohol; this is 50% of the U.S. population.

    _____ b. Cannabis is the most commonly used illicit drug in the world.

    _____ c. 75% of people with a substance abuse disorder meet the criteria for comorbid PTSD.

    _____ d. Research supports no genetic predisposition to alcoholism.

    _____ e. Nicotine dependence is the most deadly and costly of all substance dependencies.

    _____ f. Becoming dependent on drugs usually occurs suddenly.

2. Not everyone who uses drugs becomes an abuser; however, for some users, the range of chemically mediated coping responses begins with ______________________________ and progresses to ______________________________ and eventually leads to _______________ and _______________.

3. Terms of abuse are important to understand when discussing chemically mediated coping responses. Match each term with its corresponding definition.

	Terms
_____	Substance abuse
_____	Substance dependence
_____	Addiction
_____	Dual diagnosis
_____	Physical dependence
_____	Withdrawal symptoms
_____	Tolerance

Definition

a. The psychosocial behaviors related to substance dependence

b. Occurs when there is a coexistence of substance abuse and a psychiatric disorder

c. Includes withdrawal symptoms and tolerance of substance

d. Continued use of substances despite related problems

e. Severe condition (usually considered a disease) that may include physical problems and serious disruption in the person's life

f. Result from a biological need that occurs when the body becomes used to having the substance in the system

g. Occurs with continued use, as more of the substance is needed to produce the same effect

4. In addition to the history and physical examination, the assessment process includes laboratory testing for drug use. Discuss the importance of drug toxicology testing of clients who present with symptoms of possible substance abuse.

5. The assessment of a client with polysubstance abuse must be comprehensive and include key categories. List the most important areas you believe should be included in the assessment and provide one question the nurse might ask within each of these areas.

6. ____________________ is the goal for complete recovery from substance abuse or dependence.

Exercise 2

CD-ROM Activity

15 minutes

- Sign in to work at Pacific View Regional Hospital on the Obstetrics Floor for Period of Care 1. (*Note:* If you are already in the virtual hospital from a previous exercise, click on **Leave the Floor** and then **Restart the Program** to get to the sign-in window.)
- Select Laura Wilson in Room 206.
- Click on **Get Report**.
- After reading the report, click on **Go to Nurses' Station**.
- Click on **Chart** and then on **206**.
- Click on **Emergency Department** and read the report.

1. What information lets the nurse know that Laura Wilson may be abusing drugs? She was found unconscious and has a ____.

2. The assessment of chemical impairment is becoming more complex because of the increased simultaneous use of many substances (polysubstance abuse). Laura Wilson's urine drug screen was positive for THC and cocaine. Complete the table below and on the next page regarding the characteristics of these two drugs.

Substance	Route	Signs and Symptoms of Use	Withdrawal Signs and Symptoms	Consequences of Use
Cocaine				

Substance	Route	Signs and Symptoms of Use	Withdrawal Signs and Symptoms	Consequences of Use
Marijuana				

→ • Click on the **Nursing Admission** tab.
• Read the report.

3. In addition to crack cocaine, marijuana, and caffeine, Laura Wilson is abusing two other drugs. According to the Nursing Admission, these drugs are ____________________ and ____________________.

4. No drug can be considered safe when used by a woman during pregnancy. The substances used by Laura Wilson are listed below and on the next page. Describe the effects that each of these substances may have on the health of her baby.

Substance	Effect on Health of Laura Wilson's Baby
Nicotine	

Substance	Effect on Health of Laura Wilson's Baby
Marijuana	
Opioids	
Alcohol	

5. The Nursing Admission record contains information regarding Laura Wilson's precipitating stressors. Place an X next to each stressor Laura Wilson has identified.

_____ Parents' disapproval of her lifestyle

_____ HIV-positive status

_____ Unplanned pregnancy

_____ Her need to quit "crack"

_____ Boyfriend out of town

6. Select the best coping resource that is available to Laura Wilson at this time.
   a. Younger sister
   b. Boyfriend
   c. Mother and father
   d. Roommate

7. Laura Wilson's most frequently used coping mechanisms for dealing with her problems are

   ____________________ and ____________________.

Exercise 3

CD-ROM Activity

30 minutes

- Sign in to work at Pacific View Regional Hospital on the Obstetrics Floor for Period of Care 2. (*Note:* If you are already in the virtual hospital from a previous exercise, click on **Leave the Floor** and then **Restart the Program** to get to the sign-in window.)
- Select Laura Wilson in Room 206.
- Click on **Get Report** and review.
- Click on **Go to Nurses' Station**.
- Click on **206** at the bottom of the screen.
- Click on **Patient Care** and then **Nurse-Client Interactions**.
- Select and view the video titled **1115: Teaching—Effects of Drug Use**. (*Note:* Check the virtual clock to see whether enough time has elapsed. You can use the fast-forward feature to advance the time by 2-minute intervals if the video is not yet available. Then click again on **Patient Care** and **Nurse-Client Interactions** to refresh the screen.)

1. Which of the following statements made by Laura Wilson during the interaction best illustrate her lack of understanding regarding substance abuse? Select all that apply.

    _____ "The baby will help me stay on track."

    _____ "I have quit for a month or two."

    _____ "It's not like the baby will be addicted."

    _____ "It's not like I'm addicted. I can quit anytime."

2. Which of the following statements may indicate Laura Wilson's readiness to abstain from drugs? Select all that apply.

    _____ "It wasn't a hard decision for me. I am looking forward to this baby."

    _____ "I can go for a while without taking drugs."

    _____ "My mom doesn't believe I can do it."

    _____ "I'll do whatever it takes to keep my baby."

3. What do you see as the barriers to Laura Wilson's abstinence from drugs?

4. Evaluate the nurse's role in educating Laura Wilson on the effects of drug use.

→ • Click on **MAR** and find the medication ordered for Laura Wilson's pain.
- Click on **Return to Room 206** and then click the **Drug** icon in the lower left corner of the screen.
- Locate and review the entry for the medication you found in the MAR.

5. The medication ordered for Laura Wilson's pain is ________________________. In her situation, the two most important features of this medication are ____ and ____.

6. An important aspect of Laura Wilson's treatment plan will be the teaching plan. Match each of her education needs with the intervention that will best help her.

	Education Needs		**Effective Interventions**
_____	HIV-positive status	a.	Well-baby clinic and parental support
_____	Caring for her newborn	b.	Community-based self-help group and individual motivational and cognitive behavioral approaches
_____	Drug abstinence	c.	HIV counselor/HIV clinic
_____	Handling family conflict	d.	Consultation with hospital social worker/ discharge planner
_____	Community resources	e.	Family counseling

7. Relapses are common during a person's recovery. For clients who abuse substances, a key aspect of discharge planning is relapse prevention. The goal for relapse prevention is to help the person learn from these situations so that periods of ____________________ can be lengthened over time.

8. Relapse can result in a renewed and refined effort toward change and thus should not be viewed as a total failure. Discuss relapse prevention strategies you think the nurse should include in working with Laura Wilson.

Relapse prevention strategies

9. Laura Wilson will need to utilize community resources in her recovery. List four community resources you think might be helpful to her.

LESSON 9

Caring for a Client with a Cognitive Disorder

Reading Assignment: Cognitive Disorders: Delirium, Dementia, and Amnestic Disorders (Chapter 15)

Client: Carlos Reyes, Skilled Nursing Floor, Room 504

Goal: To care for a client who has symptoms of cardiovascular disease and cognitive impairment.

Objectives:

- Recognize the continuum of adaptive and maladaptive cognitive responses.
- Compare and contrast definitions and characteristics of delirium, dementia, and amnestic disorders.
- Provide examples of severe disturbed behavior associated with dementia.
- Understand underlying principles of nursing interventions for clients with cognitive impairment.
- Identify precipitating stressors associated with delirium and dementia.
- Discuss nursing interventions in working with clients who have symptoms of delirium and dementia.
- Identify underlying medical conditions that can produce symptoms of delirium.
- Identify medications used in the treatment of dementia and agitation.
- Discuss the importance of family involvement in discharge planning and home care.

Exercise 1

Clinical Preparation: Writing Activity

15 minutes

1. It is important to distinguish among the cognitive conditions of delirium, dementia, and amnestic disorders. Match each group of characteristics to the corresponding disorder.

	Characteristics	Disorder
_____	Slow development; multiple cognitive deficits, including impairment in memory without impairment in consciousness; progressive, usually irreversible.	a. Delirium
_____	Disturbance in both short- and long-term memory in absence of other cognitive impairments; always secondary to underlying causes.	b. Dementia
_____	Disturbance of consciousness and change in cognition that develops over short period of time and fluctuates during the course of a day; always secondary to another condition.	c. Amnestic disorders

2. In addition to the usual dementia symptoms of disorientation, confusion, memory loss, disorganized thinking, and poor judgment, a considerable number of individuals with dementia have secondary behavioral disturbances, including depression, hallucinations, delusions, agitation, insomnia, and wandering. Match each of the following categories of behavior to its corresponding examples.

	Category of Behavior	Examples of Behavior
_____	Aggressive psychomotor behavior	a. Incontinence, poor hygiene
_____	Nonaggressive psychomotor behavior	b. Demanding, complaining, screaming, being disruptive
_____	Verbally aggressive behavior	c. Decreased activity, apathy, withdrawal, depression
_____	Passive behavior	d. Hitting, kicking, pushing, scratching, being assaultive
_____	Functionally impaired behavior	e. Restlessness, pacing, wandering
_____	Other thought disorders	f. Hallucinating, being delusional

3. Nursing interventions for a cognitively impaired client are prioritized according to client needs. Discuss short- and long-term goals of treatment planning for a client with cognitive impairment.

4. Any major imbalance of body functions can disrupt cognitive functioning. Discuss cardiac disorders and cardiac medications as potential precipitating stressors in delirium.

5. Each plan of care for clients with cognitive disorders should reflect the

________________________________, and special consideration should be given to the

_____________________ and the _____________________.

6. In providing care to clients with dementia, the nurse must give priority to nursing interventions that maintain the client's optimum level of functioning. With that in mind, complete the table below and on the next page by listing nursing interventions that correspond to the listed components of care.

Component of Care	Interventions
Social interaction	
Medications	
Orientation	
Communication	

Component of Care	Interventions
Wandering	
Agitation	
Family and community	

Exercise 2

CD-ROM Activity

15 minutes

- Sign in to work at Pacific View Regional Hospital on the Skilled Nursing Floor for Period of Care 2. (*Note:* If you are already in the virtual hospital from a previous exercise, click on **Leave the Floor** and then **Restart the Program** to get to the sign-in window.)
- Select Carlos Reyes in Room 504.
- Click on **Get Report**.
- Read both shift summaries in the Clinical Report.

1. According to the shift reports, Carlos Reyes' most problematic symptoms have been

   ____,

   ____,

   and ____.

- Now click on **Go to Nurses' Station** and then on **504** at the bottom of the screen.
- Click on **Patient Care** and then **Physical Assessment**.
- Click on **Head & Neck**.
- Click on **Mental Status** and review the assessment.

2. During the mental status assessment, what symptoms described indicate that Carlos Reyes is having maladaptive cognitive responses?

3. Which of the following behaviors associated with aggression is Carlos Reyes exhibiting? Select all that apply.

   _____ Extreme anxiety

   _____ Irritability

   _____ Soft-spoken

   _____ Confusion

   _____ Intact memory

   _____ Disorientation

- Now click on **Patient Care** and then **Nurse-Client Interactions**.
- Select and view the video titled **1120: The Agitated Patient**. (*Note:* Check the virtual clock to see whether enough time has elapsed. You can use the fast-forward feature to advance the time by 2-minute intervals if the video is not yet available. Then click again on **Patient Care** and **Nurse-Client Interactions** to refresh the screen.)

4. How did the nurse respond to Carlos Reyes' agitation?

- Now select and view the video titled **1140: Assessing for Referrals**. (*Note:* Check the virtual clock to see whether enough time has elapsed. You can use the fast-forward feature to advance the time by 2-minute intervals if the video is not yet available. Then click again on **Patient Care** and **Nurse-Client Interactions** to refresh the screen.)

5. Assess the son's understanding of Carlos Reyes' illness. What action will the nurse need to take after her brief interaction with the client's son?

Exercise 3

CD-ROM Activity

30 minutes

- Sign in to work at Pacific View Regional Hospital on the Skilled Nursing Floor for Period of Care 3. (*Note:* If you are already in the virtual hospital from a previous exercise, click on **Leave the Floor** and then **Restart the Program** to get to the sign-in window.)
- Select Carlos Reyes in Room 504.
- Click on **Go to Nurses' Station**.
- Click on **Chart** and then on **504**.
- Read the **History and Physical**.
- Read the **Nursing Admission**.

1. Based on your chart review, what factors do you think may be contributing to Carlos Reyes' confusion?

2. If Carlos Reyes returns to his daughter's home after discharge, discuss the problems that his daughter may have in caring for him.

- Click on **Return to Nurses' Station**.
- Click on **504** to go to Carlos Reyes' room.
- Inside the room, click on **Patient Care** and then **Nurse-Client Interactions**.
- Select and view the video titled **1500: The Confused Patient**. (*Note:* Check the virtual clock to see whether enough time has elapsed. You can use the fast-forward feature to advance the time by 2-minute intervals if the video is not yet available. Then click again on **Patient Care** and **Nurse-Client Interactions** to refresh the screen.)

3. Describe the approach the nurse used in dealing with Carlos Reyes' confusion.

- Now select and view the video titled **1505: Family Teaching—Dementia**. (*Note:* Check the virtual clock to see whether enough time has elapsed. You can use the fast-forward feature to advance the time by 2-minute intervals if the video is not yet available. Then click again on **Patient Care** and **Nurse-Client Interactions** to refresh the screen.)

4. Describe the intervention the nurse used in the interaction with Carlos Reyes' daughter.

- Click on **MAR** and select tab **504**.
- Find the medication ordered for anxiety and agitation.
- Click on **Return to Room 504**.
- Click on the **Drug** icon in the lower left corner of the screen.
- Find and review the medication you found in the MAR.

5. To identify the important aspects of this medication, provide the information specified below.

Name of medication

Class

Mechanism of action

Therapeutic effect

Indication

Dosage

Side effects

Nursing indications

- Again click on **Return to Room 504**.
- Click on **Patient Care** and then **Nurse-Client Interactions**.
- Select and view the video titled **1525: Family Conflict—Discharge Plan**. (*Note:* Check the virtual clock to see whether enough time has elapsed. You can use the fast-forward feature to advance the time by 2-minute intervals if the video is not yet available. Then click again on **Patient Care** and **Nurse-Client Interactions** to refresh the screen.)
- After observing the interaction, click on **Chart** and then on **504**.
- Click on **Consultations**.
- Read the Discharge Coordinator Consult.

6. Describe the family conflict associated with Carlos Reyes' care, its implications with regard to discharge planning, and how the nurse should best approach the situation.

7. Support for Carlos Reyes' family members will be crucial for their caretaking role. Given the client's illness and his family situation, list the types of community support that you think will be most beneficial.

8. In successful discharge planning, practical recommendations are necessary for family members who must care for a client with dementia, especially those who are also agitated and aggressive. Using what you know about Carlos Reyes, provide some practical approaches below that you believe would be helpful to his daughter.

Area of Focus	Practical Approaches
Environment	
Communication	
Self-care basics	

LESSON 10

Caring for the Adolescent Client

Reading Assignment: Disorders of Infancy, Childhood, and Adolescence (Chapter 16)

Client: Tiffany Sheldon, Pediatrics Floor, Room 305

Goal: To provide psychiatric nursing care to an adolescent client.

Objectives:

- Understand the developmental tasks of adolescence.
- Identify key areas to include when assessing an adolescent client.
- Describe nursing interventions effective in working with adolescents.
- Explore unhealthy responses seen in adolescence.
- Discuss the use of a behavioral contract in working with the adolescent client.
- Explore the nurse's own issues when working with adolescent clients.
- Evaluate treatment outcomes for an adolescent client.

Exercise 1

Clinical Preparation: Writing Activity

30 minutes

1. Adolescents have several important tasks to accomplish before successfully transitioning into adulthood. What are these tasks?

2. When doing an assessment of an adolescent client, the nurse must include key elements specific to this special population. What elements should be included?

3. From the list of nursing interventions on pages 383-384 in your textbook, select five interventions that you believe are important in working with an adolescent.

4. Body image, identity, and independence are three issues that can produce a variety of healthy and unhealthy responses as the adolescent attempts to cope with the developmental tasks at hand. Match each issue of adolescence with its characteristics.

	Adolescent Issue	**Characteristics**
_____	Body image	a. Seen as being free of parental control; seeks out adult situations; can become frightened and overwhelmed in the process
_____	Identity	b. Growth and development varies widely; growth is uneven and sudden; compares self with peers
_____	Independence	c. Childhood dreams end; becomes negative and contrary; can feel isolated, lonely, and confused

5. A behavioral contract is one therapeutic tool that the nurse can use with adolescents.

   In order for a behavioral contract to be effective, it must be _______________,

   _______________ _______________, _______________ _______________, and

   _______________ by all involved.

6. Unhealthy coping responses in adolescence include a variety of behaviors. From your own life experiences, discuss the potentially unhealthy responses of depression and body image distortion of adolescence.

Exercise 2

CD-ROM Activity

45 minutes

- Sign in to work at Pacific View Regional Hospital on the Pediatrics Floor for Period of Care 3. (*Note:* If you are already in the virtual hospital from a previous exercise, click on **Leave the Floor** and then **Restart the Program** to get to the sign-in window.)
- Select Tiffany Sheldon in Room 305.
- Click on **Go to Nurses' Station**.
- Click on **Chart** and then on **305.**
- Click on and review the following chart sections: **History and Physical**, **Nursing Admission**, **Mental Health**, and **Consultations**.

1. In working with adolescents, the nurse must distinguish between age-expected behavior and unhealthy coping responses. For each issue listed below, describe the adolescent age-expected behavior. Then, based on your review of her chart, list Tiffany's unhealthy coping response for each issue.

Issues in Adolescence	Age-Expected Behavior	Tiffany's Unhealthy Response
Body image		
Mood		
Activity		

2. The specific problems of adolescence that make Tiffany Sheldon a high-risk adolescent are:
   a. substance use and truancy.
   b. severe eating disorder and depressed mood.
   c. suicidal and self-injurious behavior.
   d. problems with conduct and violence.
   e. anxiety and sexual promiscuity.

3. When working with adolescents, the nurse must understand certain basic principles. In the list of nursing interventions below, place an X next to those that demonstrate the nurse's understanding of these underlying principles when working with Tiffany.

   _____ Uses interventions that promote development of a trusting nurse-client relationship.

   _____ Lectures Tiffany on the importance of cooperating with the decisions her parents make.

   _____ Communicates empathy and understanding regarding the difficult developmental issues that the adolescent is going through.

   _____ Role-models mature interpersonal relationships.

   _____ Only meets with Tiffany together with her parents.

   _____ Maintains appropriate treatment boundaries.

   _____ Works to integrate the family's perspective with that of the adolescent.

4. Considering the psychological aspects of Tiffany's unhealthy coping reponses, discuss the type of therapy suggested by the psychiatric consultant and give a possible rationale for each intervention suggested.

5. What are your own feelings about adolescence that might arise in working with a client such as Tiffany?

6. The nurse must evaluate objectively the nursing care that has been provided to Tiffany and her family. Place an X next to each question you think would be important to consider in determining whether Tiffany and her family have met the treatment goals outlined in the treatment plan.

_____ Were Tiffany's and her parents' concerns addressed?

_____ Has Tiffany's problematic behavior decreased and been replaced with more healthy coping responses?

_____ Have Tiffany's interpersonal relationships improved?

_____ Have Tiffany's activities of daily living become more reasonable in intensity?

_____ Do Tiffany and her family have a better understanding of her problems?

_____ Are Tiffany and her parents satisfied with the progress toward treatment goals?

_____ Is Tiffany at 100% of her normal body weight?

LESSON 11

Caring for a Client with an Eating Disorder

Reading Assignment: Eating Disorders (Chapter 17)

Client: Tiffany Sheldon, Pediatrics Floor, Room 305

Goal: To provide nursing care for a client with an eating disorder who also has comorbid psychiatric symptoms.

Objectives:

- Discuss the prevalence of eating disorders.
- Identify types of eating disorders and their associated symptoms.
- Identify predisposing factors and precipitating stressors related to eating disorders.
- Assess interactions between nurses and a client with an eating disorder.
- Identify coping resources and coping mechanisms related to eating disorders.
- Apply the nursing process in caring for a client with an eating disorder.
- Develop a treatment plan for a client with an eating disorder.
- List outcomes for a client with an eating disorder.

Exercise 1

Clinical Preparation: Writing Activity

15 minutes

1. Anorexia nervosa and bulimia nervosa are the only specific eating disorder diagnoses outlined in the ____.

2. The prevalence of eating disorders is on the increase in our culture. In addition, comorbid psychiatric illnesses are common in clients with eating disorders. Which of the following statements regarding eating disorders statistics are true? Select all that apply.

_____ Only 1% of all adolescents will develop an eating disorder.

_____ 90% of clients with eating disorders are female.

_____ 40%-75% of individuals with eating disorders also have depression.

_____ The AXIS I diagnoses most closely associated with eating disorders are mood disorders, anxiety, dissociative disorders, and substance abuse.

_____ The average age of onset of bulimia nervosa is 17 years and 11-18 years for anorexia nervosa.

_____ 66% of clients with eating disorders are diagnosed with anxiety disorders, obsessive-compulsive disorders, and/or social phobia.

_____ A history of sexual abuse is less common in those with eating disorders than in the general population.

_____ Obesity is included as an eating disorder in the DSM-IV-TR.

3. Certain symptoms are reflective of a specific type of eating disorder; however, some symptoms are common to all types of eating disorders. Place an X next to the choices below that represent the most common symptoms of all types of eating disorders. Select all that apply.

_____ Intense fear of gaining weight

_____ Skipping meals occasionally

_____ Depriving oneself of needed nourishment

_____ Severe dieting

_____ Overeating under stress

_____ Chewing but not swallowing food

_____ Frequent fasting

_____ Binge eating

_____ Thinking of oneself as fat even though actually underweight

4. The psychological reasons for disordered eating can lead to which serious medical complications?
   a. Dehydration, hypokalemia, alkalosis
   b. Fluid and electrolyte imbalances
   c. Hypoglycemia, menstrual dysfuction
   d. Esophagitis, Mallory-Weiss syndrome, enamel erosion
   e. Cardiac arrhythmias, myopathy
   f. All of the above

5. How do you think the sociocultural factors related to eating disorders affect the prevalence of eating disorders in adolescent females? (*Hint:* See page 392 in your textbook.)

6. There are many factors that predispose a person to develop an eating disorder. Place an X next to the psychological characteristics associated with eating disorders.

_____ Perfectionism exhibited by rigidity, meticulousness, ritualism, and obsessive-compulsive behaviors

_____ No early childhood issues; healthy family life

_____ Pervasive sense of ineffectiveness and helplessness; no control over life

_____ Difficulty naming and expressing emotions; rapidly fluctuating moods

_____ Interpersonal distrust

_____ Inability to correctly identify and respond to bodily sensations

_____ Immaturity and compliance

7. Many people being treated for eating disorders demonstrate evidence of other psychiatric disorders. For each type of eating disorder listed below, identify the psychiatric comorbidity.

Eating Disorder	Psychiatric Comorbidity
Anorexia	
Bulimia	

8. Discuss the family characteristics that may predispose an individual to an eating disorder.

9. Do you have any sociocultural biases toward those who have eating disorders that result in being severely underweight or overweight?

Exercise 2

CD-ROM Activity

15 minutes

- Sign in to work at Pacific View Regional Hospital on the Pediatrics Floor for Period of Care 1. (*Note:* If you are already in the virtual hospital from a previous exercise, click on **Leave the Floor** and then **Restart the Program** to get to the sign-in window.)
- Select Tiffany Sheldon in Room 305.
- Click on **Get Report**.

1. Behaviors Tiffany Sheldon is exhibiting that may be indictative of comorbid psychiatric

   disorders are ________________________________, ___________________________,

   and __________________________.

- Click on **Go to Nurses' Station** and then on **305** at the bottom of the screen.
- Click on **Patient Care** and then **Physical Assessment**.
- Click on **Head & Neck**.
- Click on **Mental Status**.

2. Place an X next to each characteristic that applies to Tiffany Sheldon based on the shift report and the findings of the mental status assessment.

   _____ Good eye contact

   _____ Listlessness

   _____ Flat affect

   _____ Is energetic

   _____ Avoids eye contact

   _____ Is withdrawn

- Click on **Patient Care** and then **Nurse-Client Interactions**.
- Select and view the video titled **0730: Initial Assessment**. (*Note:* Check the virtual clock to see whether enough time has elapsed. You can use the fast-forward feature to advance the time by 2-minute intervals if the video is not yet available. Then click again on **Patient Care** and **Nurse-Client Interactions** to refresh the screen.)

3. Describe your reaction to Tiffany Sheldon's responses to the nurse who is caring for her.

- Click on **Chart** and then on **305**.
- Click on **Physician's Orders**.

4. Which of the following orders indicate that multidisciplinary assessments (in addition to physical assessments) are being implemented for Tiffany Sheldon's care? Select all that apply.

_____ Nursing supervision during and after meals

_____ Institution of an occupational therapy program

_____ Nutritionist to follow client

_____ Involvement of adolescent care team

_____ Administration of antianxiety medication

_____ Involvement of eating disorders clinic

_____ Consultation with psychiatric team

- Click on **History and Physical** and review.

5. Tiffany Sheldon's medical diagnoses are ________________________,

________________________, and ________________________.

→ • Click on **Nursing Admission** and review.

6. List at least two possible predisposing psychological and familial factors associated with Tiffany's eating disorder.

Exercise 3

CD-ROM Activity

30 minutes

- Sign in to work at Pacific View Regional Hospital on the Pediatrics Floor for Period of Care 3. (*Note:* If you are already in the virtual hospital from a previous exercise, click on **Leave the Floor** and then **Restart the Program** to get to the sign-in window.)
- Select Tiffany Sheldon in Room 305.
- Click on **Get Report** and review.
- Click on **Go to Nurses' Station**.
- Click on **305** at the bottom of the screen.
- Click on **Patient Care** and then **Nurse-Client Interactions**.
- Select and view the video titled **1500: Relapse—Contributing Factors**. (*Note:* Check the virtual clock to see whether enough time has elapsed. You can use the fast-forward feature to advance the time by 2-minute intervals if the video is not yet available. Then click again on **Patient Care** and **Nurse-Client Interactions** to refresh the screen.)

1. Tiffany Sheldon's predisposing factors make her especially vulnerable to environmental pressures and stress. Which of the following stressors have contributed to her current relapse of her eating disorder? Select all that apply.

 _____ Parents divorced 3 years ago.

 _____ Family does not understand her problem.

 _____ Mom is angry and "disgusted."

 _____ She visited her father in Florida 2 weeks ago.

→
- Click on **Chart** and then on **305**.
- Click on **Mental Health**.
- Read the Psychiatric/Mental Health Assessment.

2. Typical of those who have anorexia, Tiffany Sheldon's main unhealthy coping

 mechanism is ____________________.

3. For people with anorexia, the issue is not really about their weight, but rather about controlling their life and fears. An example of this overriding concern occurs when Tiffany Sheldon states, "____________________________________."

4. In addition to Tiffany Sheldon's diagnosis of Imbalanced nutrition, less than body requirements, identify two nursing diagnoses that best describe the psychological components of her eating disorder.

→
- Click on **Return to Room 305**.
- Click on **Patient Care** and then **Nurse-Client Interactions**.
- Select and view the video titled **1530: Facilitating Success**. (*Note:* Check the virtual clock to see whether enough time has elapsed. You can use the fast-forward feature to advance the time by 2-minute intervals if the video is not yet available. Then click again on **Patient Care** and **Nurse-Client Interactions** to refresh the screen.)

5. One of the most important factors to assess in a client with an eating disorder is the person's motivation to change the behavior. What statement does Tiffany Sheldon make that best defines her motivation level and has implications for her success in preventing relapse?

→
- Click on **Chart** and then on **305**.
- Click on **Consultations**.
- Read the Psychiatric Consult.

6. Two plans of care are being implemented simultaneously for Tiffany Sheldon. One plan involves the eating contract. The other plan is devised as a result of the Psychiatric Consult. Complete the table below to include elements of the latter plan.

Psychosocial Treatment Plan	Specific Interventions
Individual therapy	
Family conference/family therapy	
Relationship to eating contract	
Medication	

- Still in the chart, click on **Patient Education**.
- Read the report.

7. Outcome criteria are derived from the nursing diagnosis and are the expected client responses to be achieved. From the list on page 399 in your textbook, select the treatment outcomes for Tiffany.

LESSON 12

Caring for a Client in Crisis

Reading Assignment: Crisis: Theory and Intervention (Chapter 20)

Client: Dorothy Grant, Obstetrics Floor, Room 201

Goal: To provide nursing care for a client in a health crisis using crisis intervention theory and techniques.

Objectives:

- Define crisis and crisis intervention.
- Identify the goals of crisis intervention.
- Describe the four types of crises.
- List reasons for client response to crisis.
- List factors that serve as barriers to effective crisis intervention.
- Understand the steps involved in crisis intervention.
- Identify types of coping skills.
- Describe the crisis intervention strategies within each step of the crisis intervention model.

Exercise 1

Clinical Preparation: Writing Activity

30 minutes

1. Everyone who experiences a crisis can either struggle to resolve it or make the necessary adjustments to live with it. A crisis can be viewed as a _______________ _______________ with the potential to overwhelm an individual's ability to _______________ _______________, or an opportunity for _______________ and _______________.

2. Describe four types of crisis and give an example of each.

3. A person's emotional response to the triggering event of the crisis may be positive (adaptive) or negative (maladaptive), depending on several factors. List these factors.

4. List the four barriers to effective crisis intervention.

5. ______________________________ is a brief therapy initiated as soon as possible after the crisis event or crisis response. It focuses on the ____________________ problem, taking into account the context in which the problem exists.

6. Several factors influence how a crisis is resolved. List three key features that will determine the resolution of any crisis.

7. One approach to crisis intervention involves the five steps listed below and on the next page. Identify the key components of each step within the model.

Crisis Intervention Step	Key Components
Assessment of the individual and problem	
Planning of therapeutic interventions	
Implementation of interventions	
Resolution of crisis	

Crisis Intervention Step	Key Components
Anticipatory planning	

8. In the process of planning and implementing therapeutic interventions, the nurse must explore the client's current and past coping skills. Match the coping skill category to its description.

	Description	Category
_____	Worked in the past; may be remembered and tried again	a. Adaptive
_____	Sought after for creativeness and originality	b. Old
_____	Reviewed and discussed to explore benefits and liabilities	c. Maladaptive
_____	Reinforced and encouraged	d. New

Exercise 2

CD-ROM Activity

30 minutes

- Sign in to work at Pacific View Regional Hospital on the Obstetrics Floor for Period of Care 1. (*Note:* If you are already in the virtual hospital from a previous exercise, click on **Leave the Floor** and then **Restart the Program** to get to the sign-in window.)
- Select Dorothy Grant in Room 201.
- Click on **Get Report**.

1. What information in the shift report would alert the nurse that a more thorough psychosocial assessment is needed?

It is important for the nurse to obtain more complete information in caring for Dorothy Grant.

- Now click on **Go to Nurses' Station**.
- Click on **Chart** and then on **201.**
- Read both the **History and Physical** and the **Nursing Admission** sections.

2. In the History and Physical, what information indicates that Dorothy Grant may be in crisis?
   a. She is 30 weeks pregnant.
   b. Her husband beat her and kicked her in the abdomen.
   c. Her children are home alone.
   d. Her mother was beaten by her father.

3. The first step in crisis intervention is assessing the client in the five important areas listed below. In the Nursing Admission, what assessment information did the nurse obtain regarding Dorothy Grant's abuse by her husband?

Areas of Crisis Intervention Assessment	Assessment Data Found
Precipitating event	
Perception of the event	
Support system	
Coping resources	
Coping mechanisms	

4. Given Dorothy Grant's perception of the event and her coping mechanisms, what crisis intervention techniques might work best at this time?

5. Provide at least one example of how the nurse could help Dorothy Grant regain her self-worth.

LESSON 13

Violence: Abuse, Neglect, Anger, and Rape

Reading Assignment: Violence and Forensics in Clinical Practice: Abuse, Neglect, Anger, and Rape (Chapter 22)

Client: Dorothy Grant, Obstetrics Floor, Room 201

Goal: To care for a client who is a survivor of domestic violence.

Objectives:

- Define domestic violence and recognize behaviors associated with domestic violence.
- Discuss the role of the nurse within each level of prevention.
- Understand the difference between myths and realities associated with survivors of abuse.
- Discuss the role of culture in the nursing assessment.
- Discuss the use of empowerment intervention with women who have been abused.
- Describe strengths and coping strategies of a female client who is experiencing abuse or violence.
- Discuss nursing assessment and interventions for a client experiencing domestic violence.
- Identify central themes in abusive relationships.
- Understand common barriers to a battered spouse leaving the abusive relationship.
- Describe critical elements of discharge planning for someone who is being abused.

Exercise 1

Clinical Preparation: Writing Activity

15 minutes

1. Define domestic violence and describe associated behaviors.

2. Discuss the reasons that abuse often increases during pregnancy.

3. There are specific nursing interventions within the three levels of prevention. Match each prevention level to its corresponding interventions.

	Nursing Interventions	Level of Prevention
_____	Decisive intervention; if abuse is just beginning, work with couple; counseling focuses on preventing further abuse.	a. Primary b. Secondary
_____	Assist abused woman to overcome physical and psychological effects of abuse and to prevent future abuse.	c. Tertiary
_____	Identify families at risk; become politically active regarding issue, become knowledgeable about factors that increase domestic violence.	

4. There are several myths regarding survivors of abuse. Complete the table below describing the reality associated with each myth listed.

Myth	Reality
Abused spouses can end the violence by leaving their abuser.	
The victim can learn to stop doing things that provoke the violence.	
Being pregnant protects a woman from battering.	
Abused women tacitly accept the abuse by trying to conceal it, not reporting it, or failing to seek help.	

5. Discuss culture as it relates to the nursing assessment of battered women.

6. What is your attitude about domestic violence? How has this attitude been shaped?

Exercise 2

CD-ROM Activity

15 minutes

- Sign in to work at Pacific View Regional Hospital on the Obstetrics Floor for Period of Care 2. (*Note:* If you are already in the virtual hospital from a previous exercise, click on **Leave the Floor** and then **Restart the Program** to get to the sign-in window.)
- Select Dorothy Grant in Room 201.
- Click on **Go to Nurses' Station**.
- Click on **Chart** and then on **201**.
- To answer questions 1 through 6, review the following sections of Dorothy Grant's chart: **Nursing Admission**, **Mental Health**, and **Consultations**. (*Hint:* In the Mental Health section, read the Psychiatric/Mental Health Assessment; then scroll down to review the Abuse Screening.)

1. What forms of abuse is Dorothy Grant experiencing?

2. Dorothy Grant is a member of one of the special populations that are vulnerable to abuse.

   These include children, the elderly, the developmentally disabled, and ________________.

   The most widespread form of family violence is ________________________________.

3. There are general characteristics of violent families; these are listed in the left column below and on the next page. In the right column, identify any specific characteristics of Dorothy Grant's family that correspond to the general characteristics of violent families.

Characteristic of Violent Families	Dorothy Grant's Family Characteristics
Multigenerational transmission	

Characteristic of Violent Families	Dorothy Grant's Family Characteristics
Social isolation	
Use and abuse of power	
Alcohol and drug abuse	

4. What are Dorothy Grant's strengths in dealing with her abusive situation?

5. What are Dorothy Grant's coping strategies in dealing with her abusive relationship?

6. Depression is a common response by women in abusive relationships. According to Dorothy Grant's depression scale, her level of depression is _______________.

Exercise 3

CD-ROM Activity

30 minutes

- Sign in to work at Pacific View Regional Hospital on the Obstetrics Floor for Period of Care 2. (*Note:* If you are already in the virtual hospital from a previous exercise, click on **Leave the Floor** and then **Restart the Program** to get to the sign-in window.)
- Select Dorothy Grant in Room 201.
- Click on **Go to Nurses' Station**.
- Click on Room **201** at the bottom of the screen.
- Click on **Patient Care** and then on **Nurse-Client Interactions**.
- Select and view the video titled **1115: Nurse-Patient Communication**. (*Note:* Check the virtual clock to see whether enough time has elapsed. You can use the fast-forward feature to advance the time by 2-minute intervals if the video is not yet available. Then click again on **Patient Care** and **Nurse-Client Interactions** to refresh the screen.)

1. The Empowerment Model of intervention has been found to be very effective in working with battered women. The basic principles of this model are listed below and on the next page. In the video clip you just viewed, the nurse used the Empowerment Model when interacting with Dorothy Grant. In the right column below, cite specific examples of statements made by the nurse that correspond to the Empowerment Model's principles. (*Note:* If you think there is room for improvement, you may add suggestions of other things the nurse could have said to support the Empowerment Model.)

Empowerment Model	Nurse's Statements
There is a mutual sharing of knowledge and information.	
The nurse strategizes with the survivor.	

Empowerment Model	Nurse's Statements
The nurse helps the survivor recognize societal influences.	
The survivor's competence and experience are respected.	

2. The nurse uses other therapeutic responses when interacting with Dorothy Grant. These are listed in the right column below. Match each response to the technique it utilizes.

	Technique	Nurse's Response
_____	Mutual goal-sharing	a. "Feeling scared is a perfectly normal reaction."
_____	Focusing	b. "The clinical nurse specialist and the social worker work together to identify your immediate needs."
_____	Using broad open-ended questions	c. "Right now your first priority is your own well-being and the well-being of your children."
_____	Listening	d. "Would you like to talk about your concerns now?"; "Is there anything I can do to help?"

3. The immediate goal of the nurse in working with Dorothy Grant is to develop trust. In order to develop trust, the nurse must express nonjudgmental listening and psychological support. How did the nurse accomplish or not accomplish this in the video?

4. Which of the following constraints will make it difficult for Dorothy Grant to leave her husband? Select all that apply.

_____ Still in love with her husband

_____ Lack of housing and financial resources

_____ Her church's support of marriage

_____ Societal stigma

_____ Domestic violence reporting not mandatory in any state

_____ Husband in jail

5. Dorothy Grant has left her husband twice before and returned. For the battered woman, what do you think is the purpose of this behavior?

6. One of the most frightening realities Dorothy Grant may face in leaving her husband is

that he may ____.

7. Several themes expressed by women in abusive relationships are listed below. Knowing the themes Dorothy Grant is expressing will help the nurse in assessing and planning interventions. Identify these specific themes in the right column below.

Themes of Women Who Have Been in Abusive Relationships	Dorothy Grant's Themes
Lack of relationships outside the home	
Immobility to take action	
Internal feeling of emptiness	
Feeling of being disconnected	

8. Discharge planning will be crucial for Dorothy Grant. What types of discharge planning activities will be necessary for a successful outcome?

9. Discuss your own thoughts about Dorothy Grant's current and past responses to the abuse. Do you think she has responded in the way a typical person would to the incredible physical and emotional trauma? Or do you believe her responses have been more pathological in nature? Explain.

LESSON 14

Complementary and Alternative Therapies

Reading Assignment: Complementary and Alternative Therapies (Chapter 25)

Client: Kelly Brady, Obstetrics Floor, Room 203

Goal: To provide nursing care to a client with anxiety and depression, utilizing complementay and alternative treatments and approaches.

Objectives:

- Compare and contrast traditional medicine and complementary and alternative therapies.
- Define complementary and alternative medicine (CAM) and therapies.
- Discuss the trend toward the use of complementary and alternative treatments.
- List the types of complementary and alternative treatments and approaches.
- Refer clients to reliable resources on complementary and alternative treatments.
- Discuss complementary and alternative treatments for a client with depression and anxiey.

Exercise 1

Clinical Preparation: Writing Activity

30 minutes

1. The biomedical and holistic models of health care are based on different assumptions. Match each of the assumptions below to the correct model.

	Assumptions	Model
_____	Focuses on strengthening one's inner resistance to disease	a. Biomedical
		b. Holistic
_____	The scientific method of identifying causes of disease and implementing curative treatments to correct aberrant physiology	
_____	"Healing from within" or enhancing one's innate healing powers	
_____	Defines infections by the germ theory	
_____	Bases illness prevention on proper hygiene, public sanitation, and personal lifestyle choices	

2. ____________________ therapies refer to substitute therapies for conventional therapies.

   ____________________ therapies refer to therapies used in conjunction with conventional

   therapies. Together these are called ____, or

   __________ for short.

3. The greatest benefits of CAM therapies have been the promotion of

   ____________________ and the management of ____________________ illnesses and diseases.

4. It is important for the nurse to become familiar with complementary and alternative therapies. Place an X next to each statement that helps to explain why this may be true.

   _____ More than 80% of Americans use some form of CAM.

   _____ The FDA does not regulate herbal remedies and supplements.

   _____ Nursing, strongly influenced by biomedical practices, has deep roots in the holistic perspective.

   _____ Some people think treatments that are termed "natural" are harmless.

   _____ Many people who use CAMs do not check with their conventional practitioners.

   _____ Some CAMs may interfere with conventional treatments.

5. With readily available medical information, knowledgeable consumers are questioning the traditional practice of conventional medicine and turning to complementary and alternative therapies and treatments for a variety of disorders. Discuss the reasons for this trend.

6. According to the National Center for Complementary and Alternative Medicine (NCCAM), complementary and alternative health practices are grouped into domains. Provide at least one example of a complementary or alternative therapy and treatment for each domain listed below and on the next page.

Domain	Examples
Alternative medical systems	
Mind-body interventions	
Pharmacological and biological therapies	

Domain	Examples
Manipulative and body-based methods	

7. The nurse must be able to direct clients to reliable and professional information on CAMs. One organization that disseminates information on CAM to practitioners and the public is

   the ____, a branch of the National Institutes of Health (NIH).

8. In thinking about the reasons more people are turning to complementary and alternative medicine, what steps do you think the nurse could take to demonstrate a willingness to work closely with clients who may also be using CAMs?

Exercise 2

CD-ROM Activity

30 minutes

- Sign in to work at Pacific View Regional Hospital on the Obstetrics Floor for Period of Care 3. (*Note:* If you are already in the virtual hospital from a previous exercise, click on **Leave the Floor** and then **Restart the Program** to get to the sign-in window.)
- Select Kelly Brady in Room 203.
- Click on **Go to Nurses' Station**.
- Click on **Chart** and then on **203**.
- Access and review the **Nursing Admission**.

1. What two questions did the nurse ask in the admission assessment that refer to Kelly Brady's use of complementary/alternative therapies and spiritual and cultural practices? How did Kelly Brady answer these questions?

→ • Now click on **Consultations** and review the Psychiatric Consult.

2. Kelly Brady has multiple stressors in her life contributing to her anxiety and depression. List Kelly's life stressors.

3. Several conventional treatments have been recommended for Kelly Brady. Place an X next to each conventional treatment listed in the plan.

_____ Paroxetine 20 mg post C-section.

_____ Cognitive, couples, and family therapy

_____ Education regarding depression

_____ Anxiety-reduction techniques

→ • Now click on the **Mental Health** tab and review the Psychiatric/Mental Health Assessment.

4. Kelly Brady has provided the nurse with information about how she has been coping with stress. Which of the following coping strategies has she used in an attempt to deal with her stress? Select all that apply.

_____ Crying and becoming irritable

_____ Getting extra sleep

_____ Playing music and cooking

_____ Trying to go to gym or playing golf with husband on weekends

_____ Taking singing lessons and a yoga class

5. When the nurse asks her what she wants to change, Kelly Brady states that she wants better ____________________ in her life between work and home. The nurse then asks her whether she uses any CAMs, and her reply is that she has practiced ____________________ in the past.

6. There are several integrative approaches to the treatment of anxiety and depression. List approaches you believe might be beneficial in treating both anxiety and depression. Which of these approaches are found in Kelly Brady's treatment plan?

7. According to Kelly Brady's Nursing Admission, she reads the Bible and prays. Also, she has arranged for her pastor to visit her in the hospital. Discuss the benefits of prayer as a complementary therapy.

8. Based on her past attempts to control her anxiety and depression, what other complementary treatments or therapies would you recommend for Kelly Brady?

LESSON 15

Caring for the Psychosocial Needs of a Client with HIV/AIDS

Reading Assignment: Mental and Emotional Responses to Medical Illness (Chapter 27)

Client: Laura Wilson, Obstetrics Floor, Room 206

Goal: To provide psychosocial nursing care to an HIV-positive client who is pregnant and abuses drugs.

Objectives:

- Define HIV and AIDS and identify the characteristics of each condition.
- Discuss the psychologic needs of the client who is HIV-positive.
- Compare and contrast the DSM-IV-TR diagnosis and the nursing diagnosis of a client who is HIV-positive.
- List potential HIV-related psychologic problems.
- Develop a treatment plan for a client with an HIV adjustment disorder.
- Discuss the importance of family involvement in treatment interventions.
- Describe specific nursing interventions that enhance effectiveness or adaptive coping.
- Identify psychosocial teaching goals for a client who is HIV-positive, abuses drugs, and is pregnant.
- Develop a psychosocial teaching plan for the client who is pregnant, abuses drugs, and is HIV-positive.

Exercise 1

Clinical Preparation: Writing Activity

30 minutes

1. Which aspects of the social network and history of the client with HIV are critical for the nurse to assess?

2. In addition to the neuropsychiatric consequences of HIV, most HIV-positive individuals experience significant psychologic distress. The nurse who assists the HIV client with psychologic distress must understand which of the following? Select all that apply.

_____ The client and family will need help to cope with the disease itself.

_____ The client will need both education and support.

_____ The client will need guidance and support to change high-risk behaviors.

_____ Resultant anxiety and depression will take care of itself.

3. The primary DSM-IV-TR diagnostic psychosocial condition associated with clients who have HIV is ____________________ ____________________, also called ____________________ ____________________ ____________________.

4. There are many HIV-related psychosocial problems. Describe the psychosocial problems that the nurse should expect and may need to address with clients who have HIV/AIDS.

5. List five important areas to cover in developing a treatment plan for an HIV-positive client who has an adjustment disorder.

6. Families are also greatly affected by the client's response to his or her disease. Therefore after obtaining the client's consent, it is important to include family members in the interventions whenever appropriate. Which of the following family interventions would be important to include in a treatment plan? Select all that apply.

_____ Teach family members to use a problem-solving model of coping.

_____ Meet with family members separately from the client.

_____ Teach family members about the disease, its course, and what can be expected.

_____ Explain to the family that they should keep to themselves and not discuss the problems with anyone.

_____ Suggest that family members become involved in a support network.

_____ Suggest to the family that prayer is the best coping strategy for this situation.

7. After first ensuring the safety of the client and others, the nurse then focuses on facilitating interventions that enhance effective or adaptive coping to the client's multiple stressors. Below and on the next page, identify specific nursing strategies that can be used in addressing each of the listed interventions.

Intervention	Specific Nursing Strategies
Help clients maintain or improve their quality of life	
Help clients manage their feelings of fear, anxiety, grief, guilt, depression, and helplessness	
Help the client maintain self-worth and avoid a state of hopelessness and powerlessness	
Help clients satisfactorily adapt their relationships	

Intervention	Specific Nursing Strategies
Help the client maintain the highest level of functioning possible	
Help the client develop a long-range treatment adherence plan	

Exercise 2

CD-ROM Activity

30 minutes

- Sign in to work at Pacific View Regional Hospital on the Obstetrics Floor for Period of Care 1. (*Note:* If you are already in the virtual hospital from a previous exercise, click on **Leave the Floor** and then **Restart the Program** to get to the sign-in window.)
- Select Laura Wilson in Room 206.
- Click on **Go to Nurses' Station**.
- Click on **Chart** and then on **206**.
- Review the **Nursing Admission** and **History and Physical** sections.

1. Laura Wilson was diagnosed with HIV four months ago. In which of the following four categories does she belong?
   a. At risk but has not been tested
   b. HIV-positive but asymptomatic
   c. Symptomatic but has not developed AIDS
   d. Full-blown AIDS

2. Understanding how Laura Wilson might have developed HIV will determine the types of nursing strategies to be used. Discuss the possible sources of her HIV disease.

3. Laura Wilson seems to be in denial about her HIV status. From a psychological perspective, how can this best be explained? (*Hint:* Use your textbook for help with this.)

- Click on **Return to Nurses' Station** and then on **206**.
- Click on **Patient Care** and then on **Nurse-Client Interactions**.
- Select and view the video titled **0800: Teaching—HIV in Pregnancy**. (*Note:* Check the virtual clock to see whether enough time has elapsed. You can use the fast-forward feature to advance the time by 2-minute intervals if the video is not yet available. Then click again on **Patient Care** and **Nurse-Client Interactions** to refresh the screen.)

4. Laura Wilson makes several statements that indicate she is in need of significant health teaching. Record those statements here.

5. The nurse offers Laura Wilson support and education. What two specific statements made by the nurse indicate that she is offering to help?

6. How would you rate Laura Wilson's receptivity to health teaching?
   a. Very receptive
   b. Receptive
   c. Minimally receptive
   d. Not receptive at all

Let's jump ahead to review some client records not available until later in the day.

- First, click on **Leave the Floor** and **Restart the Program**.
- Sign in to work with Laura Wilson again, this time for Period of Care 4.
- From the Nurses' Station, click on **Chart** and then on **206**. (*Remember:* You are not able to visit patients or administer medications during Period of Care 4. You are able to review patients' records only.)
- Select the **Patient Education** tab and review this section.

7. Five education goals are listed for Laura Wilson. Identify the two that best pertain to the psychosocial aspects of her treatment.

- Now click on **Consultations** and review the Psychiatric Consult.

8. The consultant recommends significant health teaching for Laura Wilson. For each category listed below and on the next page, describe the specific teaching that is needed.

Health Teaching Category	Specific Teaching Needed
Support network	
High-risk behaviors	

Health Teaching Category	Specific Teaching Needed
Therapy	
HIV	
Pregnancy and care of newborn	
Community resources	